Alzheimer's Disease and Related Disorders Annual 2004

Alzheimer's Disease and Related Disorders Annual 2004

Edited by

Serge Gauthier MD FRCPC

Professor and Director
Alzheimer's Disease Research Unit
The McGill Center for Studies in Aging
Douglas Hospital
Verdun PQ
Canada

Philip Scheltens MD PhD

Department of Neurology
Academisch Ziekenhuis
Vrije Universiteit
Postbus 7057
1007 MB AMSTERDAM
The Netherlands

Jeffrey L Cummings MD

Director, UCLA Alzheimer's Disease Center
Augustus S Rose Professor of Neurology
Professor of Psychiatry and Biobehavioral Sciences
UCLA School of Medicine
Los Angeles CA
USA

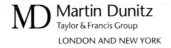
Martin Dunitz
Taylor & Francis Group
LONDON AND NEW YORK

First published in the United Kingdom in 2004 by Martin Dunitz Ltd, an imprint of the Taylor & Francis Group plc, 11 New Fetter Lane, London EC4P 4EE

Tel.:   +44 (0) 20 7583 9855
Fax.:   +44 (0) 20 7842 2298
E-mail: info@dunitz.co.uk
Website: http://www.dunitz.co.uk

A CIP record for this book is available from the British Library.

ISBN 1 84184 348 2

Distributed in the USA by
Fulfilment Center
Taylor & Francis
10650 Toebben Drive
Independence, KY 41051, USA
Toll Free Tel.: +1 800 634 7064
E-mail: taylorandfrancis@thomsonlearning.com

Distributed in Canada by
Taylor & Francis
74 Rolark Drive
Scarborough, Ontario M1R 4G2, Canada
Toll Free Tel.: +1 877 226 2237
E-mail: tal_fran@istar.ca

Distributed in the rest of the world by
Thomson Publishing Services
Cheriton House
North Way
Andover, Hampshire SP10 5BE, UK
Tel.: +44 (0)1264 332424
E-mail: salesorder.tandf@thomsonpublishingservices.co.uk

Composition by ⊼ Tek Art, Croydon, UK
Printed and bound in Great Britain by Biddles Ltd, Guildford and King's Lynn

Contents

Contributors

Roberta Anderson
PRA International
Victoria BC, Canada

C Lynn Barclay
PRA International
Victoria BC, Canada

Véronique Blanchard
Aventis Pharma
Centre de Recherche de Vitry-Alfortville
Vitry-sur-Seine
France

John Constant
PRA International
Victoria BC, Canada

Benoît Delatour
Laboratoire NAM CNRS UMR 8620
Orsay
France
Laboratoire de Neuropathologie escourolle
La Salpêtrière Hospital
Paris
France

Xavier Delbeuck
Cognitive Pyschopathology Unit
University of Geneva
Memory Clinic
Department of Geriatrics
University Hospitals of Geneva
Geneva, Switzerland

Rachelle Smith Doody
Effie Marie Cain Professor in Alzheimer's
Disease Research
Baylor College of Medicine
Department of Neurology
Houston TX, USA

Charles Duyckaerts
Laboratoire de Neuropathologie
Escourolle
La Salpêtrière Hospital
Paris
France

Olivier Guerin
Department of Gerontology (P Brocker)
University Hospital Nice
Nice, France

Deborah Gustafson
Institute of Clinical Neuroscience
Section of Psychiatry
Sahlgrenska University Hospital
Göteborg University
Göteborg, Sweden

Tzung J Hwang
Department of Neurology
David Geffen School of Medicine at
  UCLA
Los Angeles CA, USA

Vesna Jelic
Department of Clinical Neuroscience
  and Family Medicine
Division of Geriatric Medicine
Karolinska Institute
Stockholm
Sweden

Roy Jones
Director, The Research Institute for the
  Care of the Elderly
St Martin's Hospital
Bath, UK

Anne-Claude Juillerat
Memory Clinic
Department of Geriatrics
University Hospitals of Geneva
Geneva, Switzerland

Jason Karlawish
Institute of Aging
University of Pennsylvania
Philadelphia PA, USA

Martial van der Linden
Cognitive Pyschopathology Unit
University of Geneva
Geneva, Switzerland

Erich Mohr
PRA International
Victoria BC, Canada

Leonardo Pantoni
Department of Neurological Sciences
University of Florence
Florence, Italy

Laurent Pradier
Aventis Pharma
Centre de Recherche de Vitry-Alfortville
Vitry-sur-Seine
France

Magnus Sjögren
Institute of Clinical Neuroscience
Section of Psychiatry
Sahlgrenska University Hospital
Göteborg University
Göteborg, Sweden

Ingmar Skoog
Institute of Clinical Neuroscience
Section of Psychiatry
Sahlgrenska University Hospital
Göteborg University
Göteborg, Sweden

Jacques Touchon
Professor and Dean
Faculty of Medicine
Montpellier University
Montpellier
France

Bruno Vellas
Department of Internal Medicine and
    Clinical Gerontology
University Hospital
INSERM U 558
Toulouse, France

Bengt Winblad
Department of Clinical Neuroscience
    and Family Medicine
Division of Geriatric Medicine
Karolinska Institute
Stockholm
Sweden

Preface

In this year's *Annual of Alzheimer's Disease and Related Disorders* the emphasis is on the roles of senile plaques and white matter changes; interaction between Alzheimer and vascular diseases; the diagnosis of dementia in its prodromal stages, with potential cognitive interventions; trial designs and ethical issues in dementia; treatment of symptoms using the NMDA receptors antagonist memantine; management of co-morbidity; and an overview of potential diet modifications that could lead to prevention of Alzheimer's disease. This period has seen an intense interest in understanding the pathogenesis of Alzheimer's disease and identifying potential treatments. Many of these exciting developments are captured in the Annual.

This collection of chapters is an up-to-date progress report on research in the field of dementia, where advances in our understanding of causes is paralleled by improvements in study designs to test etiological hypotheses, and in our management of dementia-specific as well as associated symptoms.

The editors thank the authors for their timely and meritorious contributions.

Serge Gauthier
Philip Scheltens
Jeffrey L. Cummings

1
Innervation of senile plaques: A link between amyloid and neurofibrillary pathology?

Benoît Delatour, Véronique Blanchard, Laurent Pradier and Charles Duyckaerts

Introduction

Lesions observed in the brain of Alzheimer's disease (AD) patients may be considered under three main headings: 1) extracellular Aβ deposition, 2) intracellular tau accumulation (that is, neurofibrillary pathology), and 3) loss of synapses and neurons. Aβ deposits include a) diffuse deposits that are devoid of neuritic components, and b) focal ones, which are sometimes amyloid; that is, they are stained by Congo red. The neuritic plaque is a composite lesion, with its core made of a focal Aβ deposit and its crown composed of processes, some of which are filled with tau protein. These processes are mainly axons.[1] Microglial reaction is observed in close contact with the amyloid core[2] and is related to a low-grade inflammation.[3] Neurofibrillary pathology includes the neurofibrillary tangles, the neuropil threads, and the crown of the senile plaques.

According to the cascade hypothesis,[4] Aβ deposition, tau accumulation, and synaptic and neuronal loss are related to each other. However, the central contention of the hypothesis, the relation between the deposition of Aβ peptide in the neuropil and the accumulation of tau in the neurofibrillary tangle, is not proven. The senile plaque, containing both types of alterations, could, hence, be an important clue in explaining how they are related.

Which lesion occurs first? Which lesion causes symptoms?

From a clinical point of view, the neurofibrillary tangles are, in many studies, the best correlate of the cognitive deficit.[5–10] From a mechanistic point of view, on the contrary, disturbance in Aβ secretion seems to be essential. In familial AD, mutations of the amyloid precursor protein (APP) or of presenilin (PS, involved in the metabolism of APP) induce increased secretion of the Aβ peptide ending at amino acid 42.[11] This is also the case in trisomy 21, where three copies of the APP gene are present. In these cases, the first morphologic lesion to appear should be the extracellular accumulation of Aβ peptide. A few observations suggest that this is indeed the case.[12] In the general population, however, it has been shown that, on average, neurofibrillary pathology precedes by nearly 30 years, the occurrence of amyloid deposits.[13,14] Its progression is hierarchical, starting in the transentorhinal cortex, involving secondarily the hippocampus, and finally reaching the isocortex (the term 'isocortex' is here used as a synonym of 'neocortex'). The successive involvement of cortical areas is not due to the simple spreading of the lesion from one area to its neighbor. A spared area may be located close to a severely affected one, while it should have been lesioned if pathology had progressed by contiguity. This is, for example, the case in the superior temporal gyrus, where the lesions are numerous except for Heschl's gyri (the primary auditory area), which remain spared.[15]

Hypotheses to explain the area selectivity of neurofibrillary pathology

Sparing or involvement of a given area could be explained by its 'sensitivity' to the pathology, the entorhinal area being most fragile and the primary cortices most resistant. This possibility is contradicted by several observations: no cortical area is definitely immune to Alzheimer neurofibrillary pathology. In the severe cases, even the 'resistant' areas are affected. This implies a change in the sensitivity depending on the stage of the disease: if the 'sensitivity' hypothesis were true, a 'resistant' area would have to become sensitive in the late stage of the disease. Moreover, the selectivity concerns only neurofibrillary pathology; Aβ deposits, by contrast, are found in all areas, even in early cases.[2,16,17] Finally, the sensitivity to neurofibrillary pathology seems to be directly related, in many instances, to the neural connections. Rather than by sensitivity, we[18] and others[19–21] have proposed that the peculiar distribution of neurofibrillary pathology is explained by the connections between areas.

This relationship is probably best illustrated by the entorhino-dentate system.[20] The axons of the pyramidal neurons located in layer II of the entorhinal cortex (layer pre-alpha of Braak) end in the molecular layer of the dentate gyrus on the same side. In their way, they cross the subiculum, where they constitute the perforant path. Their endings are located in the superficial part of the molecular layer, which is made of the dendrites of the granule cells. In the entorhinal cortex, a high proportion of pyramidal neurons contain neurofibrillary tangles, but senile plaques are relatively rare. In the dentate gyrus, on the contrary, granule cells rarely contain neurofibrillary tangles, but senile plaques are abundant. These senile plaques are located in the superficial part of the molecular layer where the axons of the pyramidal neurons end their course from the entorhinal area through the perforant path. Many of these plaques have a neuritic corona. Since this corona is made of axons and since axons, in that layer, take their origin in the entorhinal cortex, one may conclude that the neurites of the plaques located in the dentate gyrus are axons from the entorhinal cortex: the senile plaques of the dentate gyrus are 'innervated' by the neurons of the entorhinal cortex. In the most severe cases of AD, the neurites of the senile plaques tend to disappear in the dentate gyrus. This is probably due to the severe neuronal loss that occurs then in layer II of the entorhinal cortex. Loss of neurons means loss of axons and of their terminal branches, leaving a band of prominent spongiosis[22,23] in the superficial part of the molecular layer of the dentate gyrus. These data suggest that amyloid deposition and neuritic innervation are relatively independent processes: amyloid deposition may occur without neuritic innervation. Loss of neuritic innervation may leave Aβ deposits devoid of axonal processes.

The possibility that neuritic pathology spreads through the connections in areas where Aβ deposition has taken place may then be raised. The following observation, dealing with an exceptional case, provides further support of this hypothesis.[24] A patient had been operated upon for a meningioma, 27 years before death. Numerous Alzheimer lesions were found at postmortem examination. The meningioma and its surgical cure had induced lesions in the frontal lobe. One small piece of cortex was massively disconnected from the white matter and from the adjacent cortices. It contained numerous diffuse Aβ deposits, but neurofibrillary pathology was absent. This observation was interpreted as indicating that loss of connections prevented the progression of neurofibrillary pathology but still allowed Aβ deposition.

Studying connectivity of the senile plaques in Alzheimer's disease

It has been proposed therefore that AD is associated with a cortical 'disconnection syndrome' in which corticocortical pathways gradually lose their morphologic and functional integrity—see reviews.[21,25] Neurofibrillary lesions could progress, in a retrograde way, along corticocortical connections from the limbic system to primary cortical areas,[18] and involve the fibers present in the plaque crown and the neurofibrillary tangles.

The fibers that innervate cortical senile plaques are mainly axons: they contain presynaptic vesicles[26] and neurofilament epitopes.[1] Some of these enlarged axons contain abnormally phosphorylated tau and, under electron microscopy, reveal paired helical filaments. Others are tau negative but are immunostained by ubiquitin: they are said to be dystrophic.[27] The pathogenic importance of dystrophic neurites (DNs) has been repeatedly emphasized.[28,29]

Senile plaque innervation from subcortical nuclei

There is good evidence that fibers from some subcortical nuclei are involved in senile plaque innervation: indeed, axons present in the senile plaque corona may contain neuromediators (or enzymes involved in neuromediator metabolism) that are exclusively synthesized by subcortical nuclei. Some axons have acetylcholinesterase activity,[30,31] suggesting cholinergic innervation from the septal area, nucleus of the diagonal band of Broca, or nucleus basalis of Meynert. Other fibers are adrenergic[32,33] and probably come from the locus ceruleus. Moreover, it has been shown in AD brains that neurofibrillary tangles develop in subcortical nuclei, such as the nucleus basalis, locus ceruleus, raphe nucleus and substantia nigra that project directly to the cortex.[34] Fibers innervating plaques originate here, as in the dentate gyrus (see above), from neurofibrillary tangle-bearing subcortical neurons.

There is no evidence of a thalamic innervation of the senile plaques. Senile plaques are rarely located in cortical layer IV[35] where thalamic axons generally end. Furthermore, AD pathology is sparse in the thalamus (except in the limbic nuclei).[36]

Senile plaque innervation from cortical areas

Senile plaques are mainly located in layer III, which contains the pyramidal neurons involved in corticocortical connections.[35] Corticocortical axons must, however, cross a relatively long distance before reaching a plaque. It is indeed exceptional to observe, in the same section, a neuronal soma and its axon ending in a plaque.

To summarize, observational data suggest that cortical senile plaques are innervated by axons coming from catecholaminergic and cholinergic nuclei. The laminar distribution of the plaques points to the involvement of corticocortical fibers, while there is no evidence that axons of thalamic origin reach the plaques.

Methods

Which tools can be selected to evaluate better the alteration of brain connections in AD?

Neuroanatomical tracing

Knowledge of neural pathways in the human brain mostly derives from old and classical methods (Golgi impregnation, retrograde and Wallerian degeneration, and myelin stains). However, modern neuronatomical tracing methods have been successfully applied, in experimental animals, to identify the neurons of origin that project to a particular brain area and, conversely, to circumscribe axonal terminal fields from a specific population of cells—see recent reviews.[37,38] Such an approach could help in decoding hodologic alterations in AD brains. However, most tracing methods rely on active axonal transport, requiring in vivo injections of neuronal tracers. Such constraints render impossible the use of these techniques to study human brain connectivity.

Despite these methodological limits, a few studies have succeeded in tracing connections in the human nervous system, in postmortem samples or in biopsy specimens that were kept metabolically functional.[39–41] However, these methods have never been applied, to our knowledge, in the context of AD pathology. An alternative approach to active transport methods involves the use of carbocyanines such as DiI (1,1' dioctadecyl-3,3,3'-tetramethylindocarbocyanine perchlorate). These dyes have lipophilic properties and can freely (passively) but slowly diffuse in the neuronal membranes, even in formalin-fixed tissue, to label cell bodies and their processes. Carbocyanine dyes diffuse in both anterograde and retrograde directions with reduced photobleaching (fading). Photoconversion from the fluorescent carbocyanin signal to a DAB staining product has also been available to stabilize tissue labeling for years. DiI tracing has been used in human brains to map local intrinsic circuits,[39,42–44] sometimes along distances that can reach several centimeters.[45] To our knowledge, the brain connectivity of AD specimens has never been directly studied with this method. Our attempts were not successful. As for active transport-based tracing methods,[46] the use of carbocyanins in human brain tissue samples has the followin limitations:

1)   The dye is transported at slow diffusion rates,[37] that is 10^{-8} cm$^2 \cdot$s^{-1}, that require very long incubation times (from weeks to months) and therefore is efficient only for short-distance tracings.
2)   Labeling efficiency is affected by long fixation times and postmortem delays.
3)   Diffusion rate is inversely related to the age of the injected specimens; consequently, the method is primarily applied to embryonic or neonatal tissue, as its effectiveness largely decreases in mature brains.
4)   Nonspecific spreading of the dye occurs in adult myelinated fiber bundles.

Plaque disconnection induced by non-Alzheimer's disease-related lesions
To clarify the origins of the processes associated with the senile plaques, we used an indirect approach.[24] By promoting selective fiber degeneration in regions connected to the lesion sites, brain lesions such as infarcts or surgical sequelae, could help to identify the neurons that 'innervate' senile plaques. We hypothesized that, if plaques lost their neuritic component following a focal brain lesion, these neurites may have arisen from the damaged region. We selected eight cases with AD neurofibrillary pathology associated with other brain lesions (mainly infarcts). Those lesions were located either in the white matter (*n* = 3), disrupting fibers with a subcortical origin, or in the gray matter of the cortex (*n* = 5), interfering with corticocortical connectivity.

In most of the cases of gray matter infarction, we showed that the cortical plaques adjacent to the lesion were appreciably denervated, indicating that neighboring (damaged) neurons were connected through their axons to the senile plaques. For instance, in one case with a small temporal cortical infarct, it appeared that plaques flanking the lesion lost their neuritic crown in a columnar way. In another case, the infarct damaged the hippocampus at the subicular level. The senile plaques found in the cortex located near the infarct lacked tau-immunoreactive neuritic processes. Infarcts of the white matter, by contrast, were not associated with a loss of neurites in the adjacent senile plaques. This suggests that subcortical inputs passing through the white matter before reaching the cortex are not the predominant source of pathologic neurites observed in the plaque crown.

Corticocortical connections seem more heavily involved in the senile plaque corona than subcortical inputs. They might play a major role in hodologic alterations occurring during the course of AD. Such results support the cortical disconnection model of AD.[21] However, these conclusions were obtained through mere observation and remain to be confirmed by experimental manipulations, which have now been made possible by transgenic models.

Alzheimer's disease and connections: Animal models

Although emphasis has recently been given to transgenic mice expressing human mutant tau and developing neurofibrillar alterations in the hippocampus that resemble human tangles,[47] most of the transgenic murine models of AD are based on promoter-driven overexpression of the human genes (APP, PS) involved in early onset familial AD that gives rise to cerebral amyloidosis in the hippocampus and isocortex—see reviews.[48,49] The behavioral phenotype of these transgenic mice, as assessed in spatial learning tasks, is greatly altered.[50–54]

Accelerated Aβ deposition in the murine model is associated with reactive astrocytosis, microglial activation, and neurodegeneration. In the vicinity of plaques, several neurodegenerative changes can be observed, including DNs. These DNs contain electrodense inclusions with dense laminar and multivesicular bodies, mitochondria, and neurofilaments, as seen in classical AD pathology. Also, as in humans, hyperphosphorylated tau-positive, bulbous-shaped, enlarged neurites can be observed in the area of amyloid (Congo red-stained) plaques.[55]

Significantly, neuronal cell loss is not obvious in transgenic mice, despite the heavy amyloid burden.[56,57] This suggests that other neuropathologic phenomena might cause behavioral disturbances. In fact, Le and colleagues[58] showed that plaque-associated neurites presented marked morphologic alterations that, as assessed by the cable-theory model, interfere with their ability to propagate neuronal information. Electrophysiologic data showing deficits in long-term potentiation induction[59] suggested that some neural networks are malfunctioning in the brain of aged, transgenic mice. Therefore, we think that the murine transgenic model, although lacking some of the classical human lesions (tangles), is suitable to investigate the hodologic alterations associated with AD pathology. We selected in vivo neuronal tracing protocols to study brain connectivity in APPxPS1 mice. To our knowledge, this approach has been used in only one other study,[60] whose authors traced the perforant pathway by injecting a tracer in the entorhinal cortex and provided evidence of abnormal, ectopic terminals at the level of the dentate gyrus.

Methodology

To test the cortical disconnection model of AD, we tried to determine to what extent the corticocortical connections in transgenic mice were altered in relation to amyloid pathology. For comparative purposes, we also investigated the morphologic integrity of other fiber tracts, namely, the subcorticalcortical connections. Ten double transgenic mice (aged 14–24 months) carrying the Swedish and London APP mutations and the PS1 M146L mutation were used for this study (Blanchard et al in press).

Biotinylated dextran amine (BDA)[61–63] was used as an anterograde tracer to visualize axonal tracts and normal or dystrophic terminal boutons. BDA is also transported retrogradely, suggesting that collateral axons from retrogradely labeled neurons could contaminate the preparation. However, we minimized the impact of reverse transport by using fine micropipettes.[63] Injections of BDA were placed at various cortical and subcortical loci.

Mice were anesthetized with a mixture of ketamine and xylazine. BDA was stereotactically injected in the brain with a glass micropipette. Tracer was iontophoresed by applying a positive, pulsed DC current. After a survival time of 7–10 days, the animals were killed and perfused transcardially with a fixative solution. Their brains were subsequently sectioned on a freezing microtome. Sections were incubated with an avidin–biotin–peroxidase complex. The following reaction made use of nickel-enhanced diaminobenzidine, which precipitated as a gray/dark product. In a second step, immunolabeling of amyloid plaques was done by $A\beta$ immunohistochemistry (peroxidase–antiperoxidase method) (DAB reaction giving a brown product) or Congo red staining.

Results

Preliminary assessment of histologic lesions in the brains of transgenic mice showed a heavy amyloid burden encompassing the allo- and isocortical regions. Plaques were also noted in subcortical regions (such as the thalamus and septum). We confirmed the existence of DNs at the periphery of amyloid deposits. These distended, bulbous-shaped neurites were immunoreactive for ubiquitin, indicating that some neurodegenerative process had occurred. At the electron microscopy level, we confirmed that numerous plaque-associated neurites undergo significant morphologic alterations.

As described below, dilated boutons containing the tracer were sometimes observed at the periphery of the plaques. These traced DNs appeared to be axonal terminals. Some neurons were fully labeled at the injection site or at a distance when they were retrogradely filled. Their dendritic tree was filled with the tracer, giving them the appearance of Golgi-like impregnated cells. The dendrites of those cells were not significantly altered in the proximity of amyloid deposits: they were sometimes rejected at the plaque periphery and avoided, in their course, the amyloid core but did not bear pathologic synapses (Figure 1.1). These data suggest that DNs are mostly composed of axonal terminals and that dendritic alterations within the senile plaques are minimal.

Corticocortical connections are disrupted

BDA was injected at various cortical loci (cingulate cortex and hippocampus). Close to the injection site, a high density of labeled DNs was observed to surround the amyloid plaques. Whatever the target cortical area, numer-

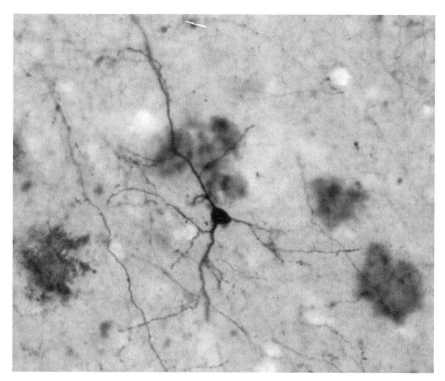

Figure 1.1

Normal aspect of neurons in APPxPS1 transgenic mouse. A neuron was retrogradely filled with biotin dextran amine (BDA) in the parietal cortex (black). The dendritic tree appeared morphologically intact in the vicinity of Aβ deposits (immunolabeled in brown). ×40.

ous BDA-positive DNs were noted at the plaque periphery (Figure 1.2a,b). These swollen, distended neurites were often observed to coalesce in grape-like clusters around plaques, as in AD.[64] Not only short corticocortical axons (such as CA1-subicular connections) but also long-distance fiber association pathways (such as cingulo-frontal fibers that course the whole caudorostral extent of the brain to reach their targets) showed marked morphologic alterations in relation to amyloid deposits.

To summarize, neuroanatomical tracings revealed that corticocortical fibers were significantly disorganized in the context of amyloid pathology, both at the local and extrinsic levels, providing a structural basis for disconnection of remote brain areas.

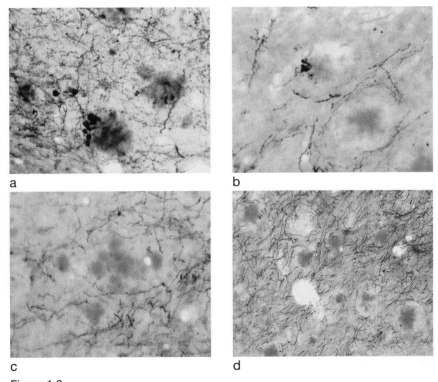

a   b

c   d

Figure 1.2

(A–B) Pathologic innervation of cortical senile plaques in APPxPS1 transgenic mouse. The anterograde tracer (BDA) was deposed in the posterior cingulate cortex. Terminal fields (black) were observed in the visual cortex (A) and in the prefrontal cortex (B). In both areas, pathologic endings (enlarged, black boutons – arrowheads) were found in the crown of the senile plaques. In panel A, the Aβ peptide was immunolabeled (white arrows); in panel B, amyloid was stained with Congo red. ×40. (C–D) Absence of innervation of cortical senile plaques by thalamic afferents in APPxPS1 transgenic mouse. The anterograde tracer (BDA) was deposed in various thalamic nuclei. Traced axons (stained in black) avoided the amyloid deposits (stained with Congo red) in the insular cortex (C), as well as in the prefrontal cortex (D). No evidence of dystrophic terminals was found (compare with panels A and B). C) ×40; D) ×20.

Subcorticocortical connections are relatively preserved

In other animals, the tracer was iontophoresed in different subcortical locations (septal and thalamic nuclei). In all examined cases, only a very small number of DNs were noticed at the level of cortical axonal terminal fields. For instance, despite very dense projections from the mediodorsal thalamic nucleus to the plaque-enriched prefrontal pole, no clear evidence of pathologic boutons was seen close to the amyloid deposits in this cortical area (Figure 1.2C and D). To confirm these observations, we immunolabeled catecholaminergic fibers in the cortex to evaluate morphologic changes in axonal terminals arising from cell bodies located in subcortical nuclei (substantia nigra, ventral tegmental area, hypothalamus and locus ceruleus) and terminating in cortical brain areas (such as the frontal and rhinal cortices). We failed to find a high number of DNs associated with cortical plaques. Interestingly, Cervera and collaborators[65] also showed the lack of tyrosine hydroxylase-positive senile plaques in the neocortex of AD patients.

While subcorticocortical connections were found to be largely preserved, we noticed that intrinsic connections within subcortical circuitries were affected around plaques. When thalamic and septal nuclei were injected, a high number of DNs were locally observed in these structures. Efferences from the septum to the accumbens nucleus and catecholaminergic fibers in the amygdala were also markedly altered in their morphology (see Cervera et al[65] for similar observations in AD brains).

To summarize, as opposed to corticocortical connections, fibers originating in subcortical brain structures did not show obvious signs of neurodegeneration when reaching their cortical targets. However, fibers remaining in subcortical networks presented pathologic endings associated with neighboring Aβ plaques.

Discussion

Results from our tracing experiments in genetically modified mice suggest that corticocortical connectivity is primarily disorganized in the context of AD-like pathology, supporting previous data obtained in human AD patients. Additional evidence could come from double-anterograde tracing experiments. The involvement of cortical inputs and the sparing of subcortical fibers could then be demonstrated in the same animal. This could be achieved by established protocols for double-anterograde tracing that are now routinely used.[66,67] An additional way to show changes in neural networks of transgenic mice would be to look for ectopic fibers[60] leaving their original targets to reach new brain locations.

Immunostaining of catecholaminergic fibers, as well as anterograde tracing, indicated that subcortical projections were not massively directed to cortical neuritic plaques. These results were also in accordance with data obtained in AD patients.[65]

However, it remains possible that some specific subcorticocortical systems that we did not directly investigate were actually impaired. This could be the case for the cholinergic system, which is severely affected in AD.[68] Bronfman and colleagues[69] showed that cholinergic fibers in transgenic mice do present an altered morphology (enlarged, distorted neurites) and constituted DNs around senile plaques—see also Sturchler-Pierrat et al.[55] However, we did not find clear evidence of axonal dystrophy at the level of the cholinergic septohippocampal pathway.

In the systems that we studied, striking differences were seen between the subcortical and cortical afferents to cortical plaques. For instance, while cingulate projections degenerated in the frontal cortex, thalamic outputs terminating in the same area showed no sign of axonal pathology. These observations suggest some kind of selectivity in the vulnerabilty of neuronal connections. Only some fiber systems are affected; others are left intact. Several factors could explain that differential vulnerability. It may depend on neurochemical properties of neural pathways. It is known, for instance, that the different neuropeptidergic systems are differentially affected, in relation to their excitatory/inhibitory properties, in the brain of transgenic mice.[70] Alternatively, one could suspect that modulated vulnerability is related to the characteristics of the neurofilaments in the sensitive neurons.[71]

Deciphering the impact of Alzheimer's disease on brain connectivity: What is the relation between dystrophic neurites and Aβ deposits?

In our opinion, axonal DNs represent a key indicator of hodologic alterations in AD. Enlarged DNs are unique to AD and appear to be restricted to brain regions with amyloid deposits. DNs are not observed in other neurodegenerative diseases (such as Parkinson's disease or Huntington's disease) that lack amyloid pathology. Conversely, DNs can be observed in Parkinson's disease with Alzheimer-type pathology[72] and in Down's syndrome.[73] Amyloidosis is present in both the latter two disorders. Knowles and colleagues[74] recently showed that Aβ deposits observed in nondemented subjects are accompanied by morphologically preserved neurites that pass through the plaques. On the contrary, the same Aβ deposit-associated neurites in AD patients show severe signs of dystrophy.

These observations suggest a close link between amyloid deposits and DNs. One might then ask whether Aβ accumulation is a prerequisite for the development of DNs or, rather, whether pathologic neurites are a primary lesion in the pathologic sequence of events.

By the amyloid cascade hypothesis, it can be proposed that dystrophy develops within neuronal processes in response to Aβ aggregation.[75] One may also conjecture that tangles, through some retrograde reaction mechanism, occur in the neurons that have damaged (dystrophic) axonal terminals.

Thus, it has recently been shown that Aβ injection in the hippocampus of tau-transgenic mice retrogradely promotes tangle formation in neurons of brain regions that project to the locus of injection.[76] It may be suggested that Aβ acts as a trophic substance to trigger pathologic sprouting of afferent fibers.[77,78] In a previous tracing study,[60] efferences from the entorhinal cortex were shown to be directed to Aβ plaques in ectopic brain locations (such as the thalamus). In that study, the neurotropic action of Aβ on axons was also observed in the white matter and in vascular amyloid deposits. DNs might equally result from some Aβ-generated neurotoxicity[79,80]—see Neve and Robakis[81] for review. Interestingly, DNs can be experimentally induced in vivo in the rat hippocampus after local acute injection of the okadaic acid toxin,[82] underscoring the possibility that DNs observed in AD result from a similar neurotoxic action. Besides the critical role of Aβ, Marcon and coworkers[83] showed that some nonamyloidogenic products of APP cleavage are also neurotoxic, and, finally, it is possible that molecular components of plaques that do not derive from APP processing also have the ability to prompt axonal dystrophy. Concerning this latter view, the α-synuclein protein, which participates in the 'nonamyloidogenic component of plaques' (NACP) and is observed in the DNs of both AD and transgenic brains,[84] has neurotoxic properties[85] that could affect neurites.

A concurrent and challenging hypothesis would be to consider that DNs are not a morphologic reaction of neuritic processes caused by nearby amyloid but do result from other pathologic mechanisms. While Aβ deposition is largely distributed in the brain of AD patients (see the first section of this chapter), the response of neurites to Aβ varies among brain regions, and senile plaques show a highly organized and restricted topography. This indicates that Aβ per se is not sufficient to promote DNs.[86] According to one hypothesis, Aβ itself is not the neurotoxic factor, but, by precipitating in the neuropil, it could immobilize local factors that would play the major pathologic role. Another hypothesis states that Aβ deposition is a late event. In transgenic mice, behavioral impairments (spatial alternation in a Y-maze) and deficits in synaptic transmission could precede the time of amyloid plaque deposition.[87–89] Once plaques are formed, some cognitive impairments (in object recognition and spatial memory) are correlated with the amyloid load,[90,91] but other behavioral disturbances are related to synaptic density, and not to the amount of amyloid deposits. Therefore, the behavioral phenotype of these mice is only partially explained by Aβ accumulation,[90] and one could easily conclude that a pathogenic event precedes plaque formation. A provocative alternative to the amyloid cascade hypothesis would be to consider that DNs promote amyloid deposition by releasing Aβ and/or its precursor in the synaptic cleft. In support of this view, it has been shown that APP is axonally transported to fiber terminals,[92,93] where it could be processed to Aβ. By means of autoradiography, APP was observed to be transported from the entorhinal cortex, via the perforant path, to presynaptic terminals in the hippocampus.[94] In the dentate gyrus, labeled APP products containing the Aβ domain were observed to accumulate at synaptic sites. In view of the observation that intraneuronal Aβ accumulation is observed before the onset of plaque deposition,[95] it is also attractive to regard extracellular Aβ as being directly secreted at the level of neuritic processes.

While it remains difficult to find out how DNs and Aβ aggregates are linked, there is no doubt that these two closely associated pathologic hallmarks compromise the integrity of brain circuitries. Disruption of cortical connections probably has a major impact on the cognitive deficit (particularly memory). The data presented here suggest that a treatment preventing abnormal Aβ metabolism and deposition should also prevent the lesions of the connective network and, hence, the clinical deficit.

References

1. Schmidt M, Lee V, Trojanowski J. Comparative epitope analysis of neuronal cytoskeletal proteins in Alzheimer's disease senile plaque, neurites and neuropil threads. Lab Invest 1991; 64:352–357.

2. Arends YM, Duyckaerts C, Rozemuller JM et al. Microglia, amyloid and dementia in Alzheimer disease. A correlative study. Neurobiol Aging 2000; 21:39–47.

3. Akiyama H, Barger S, Barnum S et al. Inflammation and Alzheimer's disease. Neurobiol Aging 2000; 21:383–421.

4. Hardy J. An 'anatomical cascade hypothesis' for Alzheimer's disease. Trends Neurosci 1992; 15:200–201.

5. Delaère P, Duyckaerts C, Brion JP et al. Tau, paired helical filaments and amyloid in the neocortex: a morphometric study of 15 cases with graded intellectual status in aging and senile dementia of Alzheimer type. Acta Neuropathol (Berl) 1989; 77:645–653.

6. Dickson DW, Crystal HA, Bevona C et al. Correlations of synaptic and pathological markers with cognition of the elderly. Neurobiol Aging 1995; 16:285–304.

7. Wilcock GK, Esiri MM. Plaques, tangles and dementia. A quantitative study. J Neurol Sci 1982; 56:343–356.

8. Morris JC, Storandt M, McKeel DW Jr et al. Cerebral amyloid deposition and diffuse plaques in 'normal' aging: evidence for presymptomatic and very mild Alzheimer's disease. Neurology 1996; 46:707–719.

9. Berg L, McKeel DWJ, Miller JP et al. Clinicopathologic studies in cognitively healthy aging and Alzheimer's disease: relation of histologic markers to dementia severity, age, sex, and apolipoprotein E genotype. Arch Neurol 1998; 55:326–335.

10. Berg L, McKeel DW, Miller P et al. Neuropathological indexes of Alzheimer's disease in demented and nondemented persons aged 80 years and older. Arch Neurol 1993; 50:349–358.

11. Younkin S. The role of Aβ42 in Alzheimer's disease. J Physiol (Paris) 1998; 92:289–292.

12. Mann DMA, Esiri MM. The pattern of acquisition of plaques and tangles in the brains of patients under 50 years of age with Down's syndrome. J Neurol Sci 1989; 89:169–179.

13. Braak H, Braak E. Frequency of stages of Alzheimer-related lesions in different age categories. Neurobiol Aging 1997; 18:351–357.

14. Duyckaerts C, Hauw J-J. Prevalence, incidence and duration of Braak's stages in the general population: can we know? Neurobiol Aging 1997; 18:362–369.

15. Esiri MM, Pearson RC, Powell TP. The cortex of the primary auditory area in Alzheimer's disease. Brain Res 1986; 366:385–387.

16. Braak H, Braak E. Neuropathological stageing of Alzheimer-related changes. Acta Neuropathol (Berl) 1991; 82:239–259.

17. Duyckaerts C, Bennecib M, Grignon Y et al. Modeling the relation between neurofibrillary tangles and intellectual status. Neurobiol Aging 1997; 18:267–273.

18. Duyckaerts C, Delaère P, Hauw J-J. Alzheimer's disease and neuroanatomy: hypotheses and proposals. In: Boller F, Forette F, Khachaturian Z et al, eds. Heterogeneity of Alzheimer's disease. Berlin: Springer-Verlag, 1992: 144–155.

19. Hyman BT, van Hoesen GW, Damasio AR. Memory-related neural systems in Alzheimer's disease: an anatomical study. Neurology 1990; 40:1721–1730.

20. Hyman BT, van Hoesen GW, Damasio AR, Barnes CL. Alzheimer's disease: cell-specific pathology isolates the hippocampal formation. Science 1984; 225:1168–1170.

21. De Lacoste MC, White CL. The role of connectivity in Alzheimer's disease pathogenesis. A review and model system. Neurobiol Aging 1993; 14:1–16.

22. Duyckaerts C, Colle MA, Seilhean D, Hauw J-J. La spongiose laminaire du gyrus denté: un signe de désafférentation observé dans la maladie d'Alzheimer. In: Besson JM, Bassant MH, Calvino B et al, eds. De la neurophysiologie à la maladie d'Alzheimer. Symposium en hommage à Yvon Lamour. Marseille: Solal, 1996: 173–182.

23. Duyckaerts C, Colle MA, Seilhean D, Hauw J-J. Laminar spongiosis of the dentate gyrus: a sign of disconnection, present in cases of Alzheimer disease. Acta Neuropathol (Berl) 1998; 95:413–420.

24. Duyckaerts C, Uchihara T, Seilhean D et al. Dissociation of Alzheimer type pathology in a disconnected piece of cortex. Acta Neuropathol (Berl) 1997; 93:501–507.

25. Arendt T. Alzheimer's disease as a disorder of mechanisms underlying structural brain self-organization. Neuroscience 2001; 102:723–765.

26. Terry RD, Gonatas JK, Weiss M. Ultrastructural studies in Alzheimer presenile dementia. Am J Pathol 1964; 44:269–297.

27. Dickson DW. The pathogenesis of senile plaques. J Neuropathol Exp Neurol 1997; 56:321–339.

28. Arai H, Lee VM, Otvos L Jr et al. Defined neurofilament, tau, and beta-amyloid precursor protein epitopes distinguish Alzheimer from non-Alzheimer senile plaques. Proc Natl Acad Sci USA 1990; 87:2249–2253.

29. Masliah E, Mallory M, Deerinck T et al. Re-evaluation of the structural

organization of neuritic plaques in Alzheimer's disease. J Neuropathol Exp Neurol 1993; 52:619–632.

30. Mesulam MM. Alzheimer plaques and cortical cholinergic innervation. Neuroscience 1986; 17:275–276.

31. Struble RG, Cork LC, Whitehouse PJ, Price DL. Cholinergic innervation in neuritic plaques. Science 1982; 216:413–415.

32. Berger B, Tassin JP, Rancurel G, Blanc G. Catecholaminergic innervation of the human cerebral cortex in presenile and senile dementia: histochemical and biochemical studies. In: Usdin E, Sourkes TL, Youdim MBH, eds. Enzymes and Neurotransmitters in Mental Disease. Chichester: John Wiley & Sons, 1980: 317–328.

33. Berger B, Escourolle R, Moyne MA. Axones catécholaminergiques du cortex cérébral humain. Observation, en histofluorescence, de biopsies cérébrales dont 2 cas de maladie d'Alzheimer. Rev Neurol (Paris) 1976; 132:183–194.

34. German DC, White CL, Sparkman DR. Alzheimer's disease: neurofibrillary changes in nuclei that project to the cerebral cortex. Neuroscience 1987; 21:305–312.

35. Duyckaerts C, Hauw J-J, Bastenaire F et al. Laminar distribution of neocortical plaques in senile dementia of the Alzheimer type. Acta Neuropathol (Berl) 1986; 70:249–256.

36. Braak H, Braak E. Alzheimer's disease affects limbic nuclei of the thalamus. Acta Neuropathol (Berl) 1991; 81:261–268.

37. Köbbert C, Apps R, Bechmann I et al. Current concepts in neuroanatomical tracing. Prog Neurobiol 2000; 62:327–351.

38. Vercelli A, Repici M, Garbossa D, Grimaldi A. Recent techniques for tracing pathways in the central nervous system of developing and adult mammals. Brain Res Bull 2000; 51:11–28.

39. Lim C, Mufson EJ, Kordower JH et al. Connections of the hippocampal formation in humans. II. The endfolial fiber pathway. J Comp Neurol 1997; 385:352–371.

40. Lim C, Blume HW, Madsen JR, Saper CB. Connections of the hippocampal formation in humans. I. The mossy fiber pathway. J Comp Neurol 1997; 385:325–351.

41. Dai J, Swaab DF, van der Vliet J, Buijs RM. Postmortem tracing reveals the organization of hypothalamic projections of the suprachiasmatic nucleus in the human brain. J Comp Neurol 1998; 400:87–102.

42. Zec N, Filiano JJ, Kinney HC. Anatomic relationships of the human arcuate nucleus of the medulla: a DiI-labeling study. J Neuropathol Exp Neurol 1997; 56:509–522.

43. Mufson EJ, Brady DR, Kordower JH. Tracing neuronal connections in postmortem human hippocampal complex with the carbocyanine dye DiI. Neurobiol Aging 1990; 11:649–653.

44. Nimchinsky EA, Vogt BA, Morrison JH, Hof PR. Spindle neurons of the human anterior cingulate cortex. J Comp Neurol 1995; 355:27–37.

45. Sparks DL, Lue LF, Martin TA, Rogers J. Neural tract tracing using Di-I: a review and a new method to make fast Di-I faster in human brain. J Neurosci Methods 2000; 103:3–10.

46. Dai J, Buijs RM, Kamphorst W, Swaab DF. Impaired axonal trans-

port of cortical neurons in Alzheimer's disease is associated with neuropathological changes. Brain Res 2002; 948:138–144.

47. Tanemura K, Murayama M, Akagi T et al. Neurodegeneration with tau accumulation in a transgenic mouse expressing V337M human tau. J Neurosci 2002; 22:133–141.

48. Borchelt DR, Wong PC, Sisodia SS, Price DL. Transgenic mouse models of Alzheimer's disease and amyotrophic lateral sclerosis. Brain Pathol 1998; 8:735–757.

49. Dewachter I, Moechars D, van Dorpe J et al. Modelling Alzheimer's disease in multiple transgenic mice. Biochem Soc Symp 2001; 67:203–210.

50. Yamaguchi F, Richards SJ, Beyreuther K et al. Transgenic mice for the amyloid precursor protein 695 isoform have impaired spatial memory. Neuroreport 1991; 2:781–784.

51. Moran PM, Higgins LS, Cordell B, Moser PC. Age-related learning deficits in transgenic mice expressing the 751-amino acid isoform of human beta-amyloid precursor protein. Proc Natl Acad Sci USA 1995; 92:5341–5345.

52. Hsiao K, Chapman P, Nilsen S et al. Correlative memory deficits, Abeta elevation, and amyloid plaques in transgenic mice. Science 1996; 274:99–102.

53. Chapman PF, White GL, Jones MW et al. Impaired synaptic plasticity and learning in aged amyloid precursor protein transgenic mice. Nat Neurosci 1999; 2:271–276.

54. Chen G, Chen KS, Knox J et al. A learning deficit related to age and beta-amyloid plaques in a mouse model of Alzheimer's disease. Nature 2000; 408:975–979.

55. Sturchler-Pierrat C, Abramowski D, Duke M et al. Two amyloid precursor protein transgenic mouse models with Alzheimer disease-like pathology. Proc Natl Acad Sci USA 1997; 94:13287–13292.

56. Irizarry MC, Soriano F, McNamara M et al. Abeta deposition is associated with neuropil changes, but not with overt neuronal loss, in the human amyloid precursor protein V717F (PDAPP) transgenic mouse. J Neurosci 1997; 17:7053–7059.

57. Takeuchi A, Irizarry MC, Duff K et al. Age-related amyloid beta deposition in transgenic mice overexpressing both Alzheimer mutant presenilin 1 and amyloid beta precursor protein Swedish mutant is not associated with global neuronal loss. Am J Pathol 2000; 157:331–339.

58. Le R, Cruz L, Urbanc B et al. Plaque-induced abnormalities in neurite geometry in transgenic models of Alzheimer disease: implications for neural system disruption. J Neuropathol Exp Neurol 2001; 60:753–758.

59. Chapman PF, Irizarri MC, Nilsen S et al. Abnormal synaptic transmission in aged APP transgenic mice. J Physiol (Lond) 1997; 501:95P.

60. Phinney AL, Deller T, Stalder M et al. Cerebral amyloid induces aberrant axonal sprouting and ectopic terminal formation in amyloid precursor protein transgenic mice. J Neurosci 1999; 19:8552–8559.

61. Brandt HM, Apkarian AV. Biotin-dextran: a sensitive anterograde tracer for neuroanatomic studies in rat and monkey. J Neurosci Methods 1992; 45:35–40.

62. Veenman CL, Reiner A, Honig MG. Biotinylated dextran amine as an anterograde tracer for single- and double-labeling studies. J Neurosci Methods 1992; 41:239–254.

63. Reiner A, Veenman CL, Honig MG. Anterograde tracing using biotinylated dextran amine. In: Wouterlood FG, ed. Neuroscience Protocols. Amsterdam: Elsevier, 1993.

64. Walker LC, Kitt CA, Cork LC et al. Multiple transmitter systems contribute neurites to individual senile plaques. J Neuropathol Exp Neurol 1988; 47:138–144.

65. Cervera P, Duyckaerts C, Ruberg M et al. Tyrosine hydroxylase-like immunoreactivity in senile plaques is not related to the density of tyrosine hydroxylase-positive fibers in patients with Alzheimer's disease. Neurosci Lett 1990; 110:210–215.

66. Lanciego JL, Wouterlood FG. Dual anterograde axonal tracing with Phaseolus vulgaris-leucoagglutinin (PHA-L) and biotinylated dextran amine (BDA). In: Wouterlood FG, ed. Neuroscience Protocols. Amsterdam: Elsevier, 1994.

67. Dolleman-Van der Weel MJ, Wouterlood FG, Witter MP. Multiple anterograde tracing, combining Phaseolus vulgaris leucoagglutinin with rhodamine- and biotin-conjugated dextran amine. J Neurosci Methods 1994; 51:9–21.

68. Geula C. Abnormalities of neural circuitry in Alzheimer's disease: hippocampus and cortical cholinergic innervation. Neurology 1998; 51:S18–29; discussion S65–7.

69. Bronfman FC, Moechars D, Van Leuven F. Acetylcholinesterase-positive fiber deafferentation and cell shrinkage in the septohippocampal pathway of aged amyloid precursor protein London mutant transgenic mice. Neurobiol Dis 2000; 7:152–168.

70. Diez M, Koistinaho J, Kahn K et al. Neuropeptides in hippocampus and cortex in transgenic mice overexpressing V717F beta-amyloid precursor protein—initial observations. Neuroscience 2000; 100:259–286.

71. Hof PR, Cox K, Morrison JH. Quantitative analysis of a vulnerable subset of pyramidal neurons in Alzheimer's disease. I. Superior frontal and inferior temporal cortex. J Comp Neurol 1990; 301:44–54.

72. Benzing WC, Mufson EJ, Armstrong DM. Alzheimer's disease-like dystrophic neurites characteristically associated with senile plaques are not found within other neurodegenerative diseases unless amyloid beta-protein deposition is present. Brain Res 1993; 606:10–18.

73. Mattiace LA, Kress Y, Davies P et al. Ubiquitin-immunoreactive dystrophic neurites in Down's syndrome brains. J Neuropathol Exp Neurol 1991; 50:547–559.

74. Knowles RB, Gomez-Isla T, Hyman BT. Abeta associated neuropil changes: correlation with neuronal loss and dementia. J Neuropathol Exp Neurol 1998; 57:1122–1130.

75. Masliah E. Mechanisms of synaptic dysfunction in Alzheimer's disease. Histol Histopathol 1995; 10:509–519.

76. Götz J, Chen F, van Dorpe J, Nitsch RM. Formation of neurofibrillary tangles in P301L tau transgenic mice induced by Abeta42 fibrils. Science 2001; 293:1491–1495.

77. Geddes JW, Anderson KJ, Cotman CW. Senile plaques as aberrant sprout-stimulating structures. Exp Neurol 1986; 94:767–776.

78. Masliah E, Mallory M, Hansen L et al. Patterns of aberrant sprouting in Alzheimer's disease. Neuron 1991; 6:729–739.

79. Koh JY, Yang LL, Cotman CW. Beta-amyloid protein increases the vulnerability of cultured cortical neurons to excitotoxic damage. Brain Res 1990; 533:315–320.

80. Yankner BA, Dawes LR, Fisher S et al. Neurotoxicity of a fragment of the amyloid precursor associated with Alzheimer's disease. Science 1989; 245:417–420.

81. Neve RL, Robakis NK. Alzheimer's disease: a re-examination of the amyloid hypothesis. Trends Neurosci 1998; 21:15–19.

82. Lee J, Hong H, Im J et al. The formation of PHF-1 and SMI-31 positive dystrophic neurites in rat hippocampus following acute injection of okadaic acid. Neurosci Lett 2000; 282:49–52.

83. Marcon G, Giaccone G, Canciani B, et al. A betaPP peptide carboxyl-terminal to Abeta is neurotoxic. Am J Pathol 1999; 154:1001–1007.

84. Yang F, Ueda K, Chen P et al. Plaque-associated alpha-synuclein (NACP) pathology in aged transgenic mice expressing amyloid precursor protein. Brain Res 2000; 853:381–383.

85. Forloni G, Bertani I, Calella AM et al. Alpha-synuclein and Parkinson's disease: selective neurodegenerative effect of alpha-synuclein fragment on dopaminergic neurons in vitro and in vivo. Ann Neurol 2000; 47:632–640.

86. Bugiani O, Giaccone G, Frangione B et al. Alzheimer patients: preamyloid deposits are more widely distributed than senile plaques throughout the central nervous system. Neurosci Lett 1989; 103:263–268.

87. Holcomb LA, Gordon MN, Jantzen P et al. Behavioral changes in transgenic mice expressing both amyloid precursor protein and presenilin-1 mutations: lack of association with amyloid deposits. Behav Genet 1999; 29:177–185.

88. Dodart JC, Meziane H, Mathis C et al. Behavioral disturbances in transgenic mice overexpressing the V717F beta-amyloid precursor protein. Behav Neurosci 1999; 113:982–990.

89. Hsia AY, Masliah E, McConlogue L et al. Plaque-independent disruption of neural circuits in Alzheimer's disease mouse models. Proc Natl Acad Sci USA 1999; 96:3228–3233.

90. Dodart JC, Mathis C, Saura J et al. Neuroanatomical abnormalities in behaviorally characterized APP (V717F) transgenic mice. Neurobiol Dis 2000; 7:71–85.

91. Gordon MN, King DL, Diamond DM et al. Correlation between cognitive deficits and Abeta deposits in transgenic APP+PS1 mice. Neurobiol Aging 2001; 22:377–385.

92. Koo EH, Sisodia SS, Archer DR et al. Precursor of amyloid protein in Alzheimer disease undergoes fast anterograde axonal transport. Proc Natl Acad Sci USA 1990; 87:1561–1565.

93. Sisodia SS, Koo EH, Hoffman PN et al. Identification and transport of full-length amyloid precursor proteins in rat peripheral nervous system. J Neurosci 1993; 13:3136–3142.

94. Buxbaum JD, Thinakaran G, Koliatsos V et al. Alzheimer amyloid protein precursor in the rat hippocampus: transport and processing through the perforant path. J Neurosci 1998; 18:9629–9637.

95. Wirths O, Multhaup G, Czech C et al. Intraneuronal Abeta accumulation precedes plaque formation in beta-amyloid precursor protein and presenilin-1 double-transgenic mice. Neurosci Lett 2001; 306:116–120.

2
Vascular factors and Alzheimer's disease

Ingmar Skoog, Deborah Gustafson and Magnus Sjögren

Introduction

In this chapter, we will review current evidence regarding the connection between Alzheimer's disease (AD) and cardiovascular and cerebrovascular disorders. The purpose of this review is to consider the role of vascular factors in AD by providing a background on vascular disease, diagnostic considerations in dementia, common pathologies of AD and cerebrovascular disease (CVD), vascular risk factors for AD observed in epidemiologic studies, the vascular pathogenesis of AD, and, finally, how AD may stimulate vascular disease.

Diagnosis of Alzheimer's disease in relation to cerebrovascular disease

Neuropathology

AD is characterized by marked neuronal and synaptic degeneration, and the presence of extensive amounts of senile plaques (SP) and neurofibrillary tangles (NFT) in specific regions of the brain.[1] Intracellular and extracellular brain deposition of the beta-amyloid peptide is an essential feature. Already before World War I, Alois Alzheimer had described changes in the cerebral vessels in AD. These include cerebral amyloid angiopathy,[2,3] degeneration of the endothelium,[4] alterations of the vascular basement membrane,[5] focal constrictions and smooth muscle cell irregularities,[6] denervation micro-angiopathy,[7] decreased mitochondrical content, increased pinocytotic vesicles and focal necrotic changes in endothelial cells,[8] and accumulation of collagen in the basement membranes.[8] Many of these pathologic microvascular changes may cause CVD or be initiated by vascular risk factors.

In recent years, several population-based neuropathologic studies have suggested that the classification of dementia disorders by neuropathology is not straightforward. First, only 50–60% of individuals fulfilling the neuropathologic diagnosis of AD had dementia or significant cognitive decline during life.[9–11]

Furthermore, several studies report that a high proportion of those who fulfill the neuropathologic criteria for AD also exhibit significant cerebrovascular lesions,[11–14] and a considerable proportion of individuals who meet the clinical criteria for a diagnosis of 'probable' AD have mixed pathologies.[11,12,15] At the same time, only minor neuropathologic changes may be detected in patients presenting with a typical picture of AD,[9,11] and the brains of a large percentage of individuals who were cognitively normal at clinical examination before death contain numerous histopathologic hallmarks of AD,[9,11,16,17] while only a small percentage are completely free of these features.[18] This implies that AD may not always present with the clinical picture of dementia. Concomitant CVD may increase the possibility that women[10] and men[9] with AD lesions in their brains will express a dementia syndrome. Furthermore, vascular pathology in AD may contribute to the clinical variability in symptoms and clinical course in individuals diagnosed with AD during life.[19] To what extent CVD contributes to the clinical picture of dementia in each case is difficult to establish at either clinical or neuropathologic examination. CVD may be the primary cause of dementia in an individual, but it may also be the culminating event that overcomes the compensatory capacity of a brain that is already compromised by AD pathology. Moreover, in many instances, a combination of minor pathologies related to both disorders may cause dementia when these minor pathologies would not have done so individually.[20]

Ischemic white-matter lesions (WMLs) are common in old age. WMLs have been described in both clinical and autopsied cases of AD.[21–25] Computed tomography (CT) studies of the brain in a population study of 85-year-olds revealed that one-third of the nondemented and about two-thirds of the AD patients had WMLs.[26] A similar proportion of AD patients had neuropathologic evidence of ischemic WMLs when examined at postmortem.[24] These lesions are associated with demyelinization and lipohyalinosis in subcortical regions, as well as narrowing of the lumen of the small perforating arteries and arterioles that nourish the deep white matter.[27] An autopsy study of nondemented individuals who had extensive AD neuropathology suggested that white-matter degeneration precedes cortical atrophy in AD.[28]

One of the most common vascular risk factors, hypertension, has repeatedly been associated with ischemic WMLs.[21,29–33] A possible mechanism for the reported association between hypertension and AD may be that ischemic WMLs increase the possibility that individuals with Alzheimer lesions in their brains express a dementia syndrome. WMLs and their associated vessel changes may also trigger the evolution of Alzheimer pathology of the brain by other mechanisms, such as blood–brain barrier dysfunction[34] or cerebral hypoperfusion.[35]

Clinical diagnosis

The typical clinical picture of AD is a dementia with insidious onset and a slowly progressive loss of memory and other cognitive functions, affecting language, visuospatial abilities, executive function, orientation, praxis, and behavior. NINCDS–ADRDA criteria[36] state that the diagnosis of probable AD requires the absence of systemic disorders or other brain diseases that, alone, could account for the dementia.

One of the controversies in the clinical diagnosis of AD is how to diagnose probable AD and concomitant CVD. Cerebral infarcts[37] and stroke[38] are strong risk factors for dementia, and ischemic WMLs are found in high proportions in both clinical and autopsied cases of AD[24,39] and may thus cause or contribute to dementia. A diagnosis of vascular dementia (VAD) will often be assigned if a patient has a history of CVD; thus, dementias will often be classified on the basis of the presence or absence of stroke. There is, however, a clinical overlap between AD and VAD.[40] These disorders may present with similar symptomatology,[41–43] a fact which also is reflected in current diagnostic criteria, such as those of DSM-IV, where the symptomatic criteria for AD and VAD are identical, except regarding the presence or absence of CVD.[44] The complexity of the diagnosis is further emphasized by the fact that patients with the neuropathologic diagnosis of VAD often present with an insidious onset and a slowly progressive course without focal signs or infarcts on brain imaging (especially when CT has been used).[45] In addition, several biological markers of AD, such as increased tauprotein[46] and decreased beta-amyloid levels [47] in cerebrospinal fluid (CSF), may be observed in VAD; and markers for CVD, such as an increased ratio of CSF albumin to blood albumin[34] indicating blood–brain barrier dysfunction, are often seen in AD. Finally, similar patterns of cerebral blood-flow changes are reported in AD and VAD, further underscoring the overlap between these disorders.[48]

Another problem in the diagnosis is that CVD is often unrecognized in individuals diagnosed with AD. Unrecognized CVD may be especially common in higher ages, as the frequency of silent infarcts increases with age,[49] and silent infarcts are related to an increased incidence of dementia.[37] Poststroke dementia is probably a mixture of the direct consequences of stroke, pre-existing AD pathology, and the additive effects of these lesions and the aging processes.[50] All these data support the notion that these two disorders, which are thought to be distinct and separate, may coexist, and aggravate and induce each other.[50] The complexity of the diagnosis in cases with mixed pathology may be one reason why the use of different diagnostic criteria for VAD results in substantial differences in the proportion of demented individuals diagnosed with VAD or AD.[41,51,52]

It has also been suggested that individuals with AD may be at increased risk of stroke and cerebral infarction. Two studies[53,54] reported that elderly individuals without previous stroke and with very low cognitive ability were at increased risk of the later development of stroke. A third study reported that both mild cognitive impairment and mild dementia were associated with an increased incidence of new strokes.[55] Even if the clinical manifestations of AD may increase the risk of later stroke, it is not clear whether the neuropathologic features of AD and cerebral infarcts are associated.[10]

Cardiovascular risk factors and Alzheimer's disease

Established risk factors for AD include age, Down's syndrome, low educational level, family history of dementia, and female gender after age 80.[56] In the 1990s, numerous epidemiologic and autopsy studies reported associations between CVD risk factors, such as hypertension,[29,57,58] high cholesterol levels,[58,59] obesity[60] and diabetes mellitus,[61,62] and the neuropathologic and clinical manifestations of AD.[63,64] These vascular factors often occur together; fewer than 20% occur in isolation.[65] This clustering is often attributed to an insulin-resistance syndrome promoted by abdominal obesity or the metabolic cardiovascular syndrome. Risk of CVD increases with the extent of risk-factor clustering.[65] For example, only 14% of coronary events in hypertensive men and 5% of those in hypertensive women occurred in the absence of additional risk factors in the Framingham Study.[65] It is not clear whether the same is true of the relation between vascular factors and AD, but the metabolic cardiovascular syndrome has been related to dementia,[66] and features of the insulin-resistance syndrome have been associated with AD.[67] However, although high cholesterol levels and hypertension often cluster, these two entities seem to be independent risk factors for AD.[59] In further support of an association between AD and vascular factors, one established vulnerability gene for vascular disease, apolipoprotein E4 (APOE), is also a vulnerability gene for AD.

Hypertension

Hypertension is currently defined as systolic blood pressure (SBP) above 160 mmHg and/or diastolic blood pressure (DBP) above 90 mmHg, but the threshold for hypertension has decreased in recent years. The incidence of hypertension increases with age.[68] Hypertension is a risk factor for stroke, ischemic WMLs, silent infarcts, general atherosclerosis, myocardial infarction, and cardiovascular morbidity and mortality.[65]

During the 1990s, evidence accumulated that hypertension may also be a risk factor for cognitive decline and dementia, independent of the presence of CVD. Hypertension has been found to be associated with brain load of SP and NFT, that is, the neuropathologic hallmarks of AD. In the Honolulu–Asia Aging Study, an elevated midlife SBP (160 mmHg or above) was found to be associated with lower brain weight and greater numbers of SP in both neocortex and hippocampus,[69] and DBP elevation (95 mmHg or above) was associated with greater numbers of NFT in the hippocampus. It is possible that this pathologic relationship develops early in the course of the disease, that is, before the onset of dementia, since an increased amount of NFT and SP has been observed in the autopsied brains of nondemented, middle-aged individuals with hypertension.[70]

Hypertension has also been associated with the clinical manifestations of AD. Several longitudinal studies have examined the association between blood pressure and dementia. Most of these suggest an association between AD and hypertension,[29,57,58,71–73] although some do not.[74–77] Some of these latter studies, however, reported an association with vascular dementia.[74,75,77] A common feature of studies reporting an association between hypertension and AD is a long observation time of follow-up before the onset of dementia. The first report from a longitudinal study showed that both high SBP and high DBP preceded the onset of clinical AD by 10–15 years.[29] This finding was verified in the Honolulu–Asia Aging Study, in which 3703 Japanese-American men were examined during 1965–71, and re-examined for dementia in 1991. In this study, a high SBP (above 160 mmHg) or high DBP (above 90 mmHg) predicted the diagnosis of AD and VAD 20–26 years later.[57] A Finnish study reported that high SBP (above 160 mmHg) in midlife predicted the diagnosis of AD 20 years later.[58] The latest follow-up in the Rotterdam Study[72] reported that high blood pressure precedes AD by approximately 9 years. In a recent report from the 6-year follow-up of the Kungsholmen Study, high SBP (above 180 mmHg), and low DBP (below 140 mmHg) were related to an increased incidence of AD.[71] The authors argued that pulse pressure may be important.[78] All these reports suggest that hypertension as a risk factor for AD appears many years before the onset of the disease.

The risk of cardiovascular events increases with increasing blood pressure also at blood pressure within the normal ranges,[65] and a high percentage of these cardiovascular events occur in those with normal blood pressure or mild hypertension.[79] For example, one-fourth of the events in elderly women and one-third in elderly men in the Framingham Study occurred in persons who had SBP of 140–159 mmHg and/or 90–95 mmHg DBP.[65] The same pattern may be true for AD, as the risk of developing dementia increased with increasing blood pressure at baseline, even within the lower ranges of observed blood pressures in the Gothenburg Longitudinal Study on Aging.[29]

Cross-sectional studies and studies with short follow-ups provide a different picture of the blood pressure–dementia relationship compared with long-term prospective studies. Cross-sectional studies[80–82] and studies with short follow-ups[83,84] have consistently reported associations between low blood pressure and prevalent or incident AD. Medium-long follow-up studies sometimes report that both high and low blood pressures are related to the incidence of AD.[71]

There are several explanations for the association between low blood pressure and AD. Skoog et al[29] reported that blood pressure decreases in the years preceding AD onset, and others have reported that blood pressure declines during the course of AD[85,86] and with increasing dementia severity.[80,81] The strength of the low blood pressure–dementia relationship was explored in a longitudinal study where low blood pressure was related to a low Mini-Mental State Examination (MMSE) score at baseline, but not to incident AD when controlling for baseline MMSE.[84] The low blood pressure observed during preclinical and manifest dementia is probably due to the brain lesions in manifest and preclinical AD. The hypothalamus, amygdala, insular cortex, medial prefrontal cortex, locus ceruleus, parabrachial nucleus, pons, and medulla oblongata are involved in central blood pressure regulation,[85,87,88] and several of these brain regions are affected in AD.[89] For example, a strong correlation was observed between the number of C-1 neurons in the medulla oblongata and blood pressure in AD patients in one study;[85] in another study, brain atrophy was associated with lower blood pressure in both demented and nondemented 85-year-olds.[81]

Low blood pressure is probably a secondary event in the development of AD, but may in itself aggravate the disease, as a spectrum of ischemic neuronal brain lesions[90] and loss of myelin in the white matter[21] may occur when systemic hypotension is accompanied by reduced cerebral blood flow. Reduction in cerebral blood flow[86] and progressive development of cerebral hypoperfusion[35] has therefore been suggested to play a role in the pathogenesis of AD.

Treatment of hypertension

Treatment of hypertension has been proven to reduce cardiovascular risk substantially in the elderly, but a large proportion of hypertensive people are not treated. Observational studies report that users of antihypertensive drugs seem to have a lower incidence of AD than nonusers.[91] One study showed that individuals who developed dementia between the ages of 79 and 85 used fewer antihypertensive drugs between the ages of 70 and 79 than those who did not develop dementia.[29] This protective effect of antihypertensive treatment may be especially evident in carriers of the APOE $\varepsilon 4$ allele.[92] Other observational studies have been less conclusive, with nonsignificant odds ratios below 1.00 for risk of AD,[93,94] although the latter study showed a significant protective effect for overall dementia. In the Honolulu–Asia Aging Study, the association between hypertension and the development of AD was strongest among men who were never treated for hypertension.[57]

Regarding placebo-controlled trials, the Syst-Eur study[95] reported that treatment of isolated systolic hypertension (SBP > 165 mmHg and DBP < 95 mmHg) with the long-acting calcium channel blocker, nitrendipine, reduced the incidence of dementia (mainly AD) by 50%. However, only 11 individuals in the nitrendipine group and 22 in the placebo group developed dementia. All randomized patients in Syst-Eur were offered active study medication for a further period of observation, which increased follow-up to 3.9 years and the total number of dementia cases to 64 (64% AD).[96] Those on active treatment during the double-blind phase of the study continued to have a lower blood pressure than the controls, and had a 55% reduced risk of dementia during the extended follow-up. This study and other antihypertensive trials[97,98] suggest that treatment of hypertension does not increase dementia risk in the elderly.

Apolipoprotein E

The ε4 allele of APOE has been associated with coronary heart disease,[99,100] atherosclerosis,[101] and hypercholesterolemia,[102] and is an established susceptibility gene for both the neuropathologic[103] and clinical manifestations of AD.[104–106] Interactions between the APOE ε4 genotype and vascular diseases, such as generalized atherosclerosis[107] and ischemic WMLs,[108] affecting the risk of AD have also been reported.

Apolipoprotein E is an essential ligand for the transport and redistribution of lipids,[109] mainly triglyceride-rich, very-low-density lipoproteins (VLDL) and cholesterol-enriched remnant lipoproteins. An important property of apolipoprotein E is its ability to mediate the binding of these lipoproteins to the low-density lipoprotein (LDL) receptor and to the LDL-receptor-related protein (LRP).[110] LDL is the main carrier of cholesterol in the blood and is considered to be the most atherogenic of the plasma lipoproteins[111] and the most closely associated with coronary artery disease.[112] Apolipoprotein E may also be involved in the injury–repair response in the artery wall, and thus in the progression and regression of atherosclerotic lesions.[109] Apolipoprotein E is also present in the brain, where it is known to have a general repair function.[109] APOE ε4 inheritance may also have a direct effect on β-amyloid pathology, as APOE transgenic or knockout mice show reduced deposition of β-amyloid.[113] APOE ε4 also binds with high avidity to β-amyloid peptides and enhances the formation of β-amyloid fibrils.[114]

Blood cholesterol

Elevation in plasma cholesterol, particularly the proportion carried by LDL, is linked to atherosclerosis and is also often elevated in individuals with hypertension. Late-life high-density lipoprotein (HDL) cholesterol and, to a certain extent, midlife HDL cholesterol were associated with the amount of neocortical and hippocampal SP and neocortical NFT in the Honolulu–Asia Study.[115] Furthermore, cholesterol located in the brain cortex has been found to be increased in both coronary heart disease and AD.[116] The clinical manifestations of AD have also been associated with high cholesterol. Two Finnish studies reported that individuals with AD had high cholesterol levels 15–30 years before disease onset.[58,117] It has been suggested that the effect of APOE on the risk of AD may be partially mediated through high serum cholesterol levels. However, in both the Honolulu–Asia Study[115] and the study by Kivipelto et al,[59] the effect of cholesterol on AD manifestations was independent of the APOE ε4 allele. There is additional evidence of a relation between cholesterol and AD. A cholesterol-rich diet results in an increased intensity of apolipoprotein E immunoreactivity in neurons,[118] suggesting that elevated circulating levels of blood cholesterol may result in increased cerebral levels.

Treatment of hypercholesterolemia

Statins, such as lovastatin and simvastatin, are used to lower high cholesterol levels in humans. Adding lovastatin to cellular cultures reduces the conversion of APP to Abeta.[119] In a more recent study, simvastatin and lovastatin reduced intracellular and extracellular levels of Abeta-42 and Abeta-40 in primary cultures of hippocampal neurons and mixed cortical neurons.[120] Furthermore, guinea pigs treated with high doses of simvastatin showed a strong and reversible reduction of Abeta-42 and Abeta-40 levels in CSF and in brain homogenate. One study also found that feeding transgenic AD mice a diet high in cholesterol increased the production of neuritic plaques, while statin treatment (atorvastatin) reduced the production of neuritic plaques by approximately 50%.[121,122] In support of the hypothesis that statins may prevent AD, two case record-based studies reported a reduced frequency of dementia[123] and AD[124] in statin-treated individuals. However, case-record studies have many methodological problems in studying AD, such as underdetection and indication-for-treatment bias. The recent longitudinal observation from the Canadian Study of Health and Aging[125] that the incidence of AD was reduced in individuals using statins further supports the hypothesis that cholesterol may be important in AD.

Hitherto, two clinical prospective trials have been performed. In a double-blind, placebo-controlled randomized trial, 44 patients with AD were studied for the possible effect of simvastatin treatment. Both clinical and biochemical measures were investigated. After 26 weeks of treatment, no difference in either psychometric or biochemical measures were found, but a post hoc analysis revealed a slight reduction in the CSF levels of Aβ40 ($P < 0.05$) in mildly demented patients.[126] In a second study, 19 patients with AD were treated in an open trial with 20 mg simvastatin for 12 weeks. After 12 weeks, the CSF levels of α-secretase-cleaved APP and β-secretase-cleaved APP were found to be significantly reduced ($P < 0.001$), but the CSF levels of tau, phospho-tau, and Aβ42 and the plasma levels of Aβ were unchanged. The ADAS-cog score was slightly increased ($P < 0.05$). The results of this study suggest that simvastatin acts directly on the processing of APP by inhibiting both the α- and the β-secretase pathways.[127] However, since both these studies followed patients who already had AD, and for a rather short time period, future studies must follow AD patients for a longer time, and initiate treatment at an early stage or even before the manifestations of the disease.

Diabetes mellitus

A report from the Honolulu–Asia Aging Study, including 216 subjects who underwent autopsy, found that participants with type 2 diabetes and the ϵ4 allele had an increased number of hippocampal neuritic plaques (NP) and NFT in the cortex and hippocampus, and they had a higher risk of cerebral amyloid angiopathy.[128]

The clinical manifestations of AD have also been related to diabetes mellitus. In the 2-year follow-up of the Rotterdam Study, diabetes mellitus at baseline almost doubled the risk of incident AD.[62] The highest risk was observed among patients treated with insulin. Type 2 diabetes was also associated with increased incidence of AD in the Rochester medical records database.[129] In contrast, after multivariate adjustment, the Honolulu–Asia Aging Study reported no association between AD and diabetes that was present either 25 or 15 years prior to AD diagnosis.[130] A significant association was, however, found between impaired glucose tolerance at baseline and incidence of VAD. A later report from the Honolulu–Asia Aging Study, including 216 subjects who underwent autopsy, found that type 2 diabetes was associated with incidence of total dementia, AD, and VAD.[128] A Finnish study reported a cross-sectional association between AD and features of the insulin-resistance syndrome.[67] The association between AD and diabetes mellitus is not completely clear, as several incidence studies did not find an association between AD and diabetes mellitus.[77,131,132] Instead, all these studies reported that diabetes mellitus was a risk factor for VAD.

There are several potential pathways by which diabetes may lead to AD. Diabetes is associated with changes in the blood–brain barrier and with the transport function of cerebral microvessels.[133] Diabetes is also accompanied by an increased oxidative stress and formation of advanced glycation end products (AGE). These AGE deposit in tissues and contribute to the diabetic microvascular complications[134] such as increased atherogenesis.[135] The receptor for AGE (RAGE),[136] which is found on the surface of neurons, microglia, and vascular endothelium, is also activated by Abeta,[136] leading to increased accumulation of AGE. Increased AGE leads to prolonged half-life of Abeta and also to increased accumulation of Abeta.[137] Thereby, a vicious cycle may be turned on, involving Abeta and AGE. Furthermore, insulin regulates phosphorylation of tau protein, and affects the metabolism of beta-amyloid.[61,138]

CNS dysfunction in diabetes may also be mediated through other diabetes-related conditions, such as hypertension; obesity; decreased peripheral circulation; ischemia; uremia; peripheral and autonomic neuropathy; the use of multiple drugs; other neuroendocrine or neurochemical changes; and the consequences of hyper- and hypoglycemia, hyperinsulinemia, and ketoacidosis.[139]

Coronary heart disease and atherosclerosis

There is also evidence that coronary heart disease and atherosclerosis are related to AD. For example, myocardial infarction has been associated with increased incidence of AD in women[140] and with increased amounts of senile plaques in two autopsy studies.[141,142] Furthermore, atrial fibrillation[143] and generalized atherosclerosis[107] have been associated with the clinical manifestations of AD in cross-sectional analyses. Atrial fibrillation[144,145] and carotid atherosclerosis[146] have been associated with WMLs and silent infarcts, which may contribute to impairment of cognitive function, and also lead to cerebral hypoperfusion, one of the putative important pathophysiological mechanisms of AD.[35] In this respect, the process may be further aggravated by concomitant hypertension and high cholesterol levels, which are risk factors for both myocardial infarction and atherosclerosis, as well as independent risk factors for AD.

Putative shared pathogenetic mechanisms in Alzheimer's disease and vascular dementia

The association between AD and vascular factors may be mediated through different pathogenetic pathways, such as oxidative stress, ischemia, blood–brain barrier dysfunction, apoptosis, disturbance in the renin–angiotensin system (RAS), and psychological stress. The associations may go in different directions; vascular disease may cause or exacerbate AD pathology, AD pathology may cause or exacerbate CVD, or both may share similar pathogenetic pathways.

Oxidative stress

There is strong support for the involvement of oxidative stress and the formation of free radicals in vascular disorders, such as atherosclerosis, early hypertension, myocardial infarction, diabetes mellitus, and stroke, and also in AD.[147] In AD, Abeta induces oxidative stress in neurons[136,148] and interacts with endothelial cells to produce an excess of free radicals.[149] Activation generates reactive oxygen species, which in combination with lower activities of antioxidant enzymes such as superoxide dismutase and catalase, may lead to damage to the endothelium[150] and neurons.[136] Furthermore, AD and VAD patients have a disturbance in protective antioxidant systems, which may make them even more vulnerable to oxidative stress.[151] Taken together, activation of oxidative stress may induce a self-perpetuating process that is a major part of the degenerative process in AD.

Ischemia

Ischemia may influence the pathogenesis of AD.[152] Several experimental studies on animals suggest that ischemia may lead to accumulation of APP and Abeta.[153–156] Ischemia may also influence the expression of the presenilin,[157,158] which may lead to an increase in Abeta-42.[159,160] Ischemia may also accelerate the pathogenesis of AD through the formation of oxygen radicals.[161] There is also a possibility that Alzheimer encephalopathy may exacerbate neuronal damage after ischemia.[162]

Blood–brain barrier dysfunction

Under normal conditions, the tight junctions, the absence of fenestrations, and the paucity of pinocytosis in brain capillary endothelium act as an effective barrier between the brain and circulating toxic agents, components of the immune system, proteins, breakdown products, or brain-directed antibodies.[163] This blood–brain barrier (BBB) comprises the major diffusion barrier between the blood and the brain. Hypertension[164–167] and diabetes mellitus[133] may lead to a disturbance in the BBB. A BBB dysfunction has been suggested to be involved in the etiology and pathogenesis of AD.[168–170] The CSF albumin to serum albumin ratio is a method of assessing the BBB function in living subjects. BBB dysfunction in AD has been supported by some CSF studies,[34,171–173] but not others.[174–176] A mild BBB dysfunction may increase the possibility that substances from serum penetrate the BBB and reach the brain, where they may interact with neurons,[168] leading to inflammation or perhaps starting a cascade of amyloid accumulation and Alzheimer encephalopathy.

The renin–angiotensin system

The RAS may be involved in both vascular diseases and in AD. The active octapeptide angiotensin II is produced by conversion of the largely inactive angiotensin I by the angiotensin I-converting enzyme (ACE).[177] Angiotensin II has a number of effects on the cardiovascular system, including direct vasoconstriction, aldosterone secretion stimulation, sodium retention, sympathetic nervous system activation,[177] and promotion of hyperplasia and hypertrophy in vascular smooth muscle cells.[178] The findings that treatment with ACE inhibitors reduces hypertrophy of cremaster arterioles and prevents remodeling of cerebral arterioles in stroke-prone, spontaneously hypertensive rats,[179] and that treatment with ACE inhibitors normalizes the structure of peripheral arteries in hypertensive patients[180] may have implications for AD in view of the possible role of WMLs and microvascular changes in this disorder.

   The RAS is also active in the brain, as in regulation of behavioral and physiologic responses, such as central tonic blood pressure control and cerebral blood-flow autoregulation.[181] In experimental models of cognitive function, elevated levels of angiotensin II impair learning, especially acquisition and recall of newly learned material, and other memory functions.[181,182] Angiotensin II receptor antagonists[183] and ACE inhibitors[181] improve cognitive function in mice. Furthermore, an increased activity of the ACE in different areas of the brain has been reported in AD patients.[184,185] These findings suggest that the RAS system may be involved in the pathogenesis and clinical expression of AD.

Lifestyle and psychological stress

Early traumatic life events have been associated with hypertension[186] with an increased incidence of AD.[187] Stress during neonatal handling in rats increases glucocorticoid levels, and may lead to impairment of the hippocampus,[188,189] a brain region that is impaired early in AD. Some lifestyle factors suggested to protect against cardiovascular disorders, such as use of estrogen,[190] moderate consumption of red wine,[191] and use of antioxidants,[192] may protect against AD and may modify the pathogenesis of the disorder.

Smoking is a strong risk factor for vascular diseases, such as hypertension, atherosclerosis, coronary heart disease, and diabetes mellitus. However, despite recent associations found between vascular diseases and AD, the association between smoking and AD is less clear. In cross-sectional studies, smoking is often associated with a low frequency of AD,[193,194] while the results from longitudinal studies are conflicting. In the Rotterdam Study, current smoking increased the incidence of dementia and AD among carriers of the APOE ε4 allele,[195] and a pooled analysis of four European population-based prospective studies of individuals 65 years and older also showed smoking to be a risk factor for AD.[196] However, no association in any direction was reported from other follow-up studies.[197,198] While increased risk of AD in smokers may be related to vascular factors, a possible inverse relationship may be explained by the possibility that smoking increases the density of cholinergic nicotine receptors in the brain.[193] These contrasting physiologic effects of smoking may explain the inconsistent reports on the relationship between AD and smoking.

Alzheimer's disease stimulating vascular disease

Initiation and/or progression of vascular disease may also be a consequence of AD. The interaction of Abeta with endothelial cells of rat aorta produces an excess of superoxide radicals. This process led to damage of the endothelium. It also scavenged the endothelium-derived relaxing factor (EDRF), leading to enhanced vasoconstriction.[149] EDRF maintains the vasculature in a constant state of vasodilation, due to continuous release of endothelial nitric oxide (eNO).[199] Inhibition of eNO release leads to acute and sustained hypertension.[200]

Serum Abeta levels are elevated in some forms of familial AD, as well as in some sporadic AD cases. Intra-arterial soluble Abeta infusions in animals increase vascular resistance in the cerebral cortex,[201] impair BBB function,[202] and increase mean arterial blood pressure compared with vehicle distilled water infusion.[203] Circulating Abeta-40 may thus exert vasopressor actions in vivo that precede Abeta deposition and dementia onset, and may be one reason for the observed association between previous high blood pressure and AD.

Conclusion

The reported association between AD and vascular diseases may teach us more about the pathogenesis of the disorder, but it also has implications for the clinical management of AD and cardiovascular disease. While it appears clear that there is an association between AD and vascular factors, the exact mechanism behind this association is far from clear. There are, however, several possible explanations: silent CVD may be overlooked in AD but may increase the likelihood that individuals with AD changes in their brain will express a dementia syndrome, vascular factors may stimulate the AD process, AD may stimulate the evolution of vascular disorders, and similar biologic mechanisms may be involved in the pathogenesis of both vascular disorders and AD.[61,64]

The association between AD and vascular diseases has several clinical implications. It is important to search for treatable cardiovascular disease and CVD in the evaluation of AD patients, as these may influence the expression and clinical manifestations of the disease. It is also important to detect cognitive impairment in patients with cardiovascular diseases, as cognitive dysfunction in these patients has implications for the management and may decrease patients' compliance with treatment. Patients with concomitant AD and CVD may also benefit from treatment with acetylcholinesterase inhibitors.[204]

Vascular disorders and risk factors are common in the elderly and therefore are important targets in the prevention of dementia. Thus, even if they result in only a moderately increased risk of AD or overall dementia, they may have an immense effect on the total number of affected individuals.[205]

Acknowledgments

The work was supported by a grant from the Swedish Research Council for Social Sciences (project no. 0914), and the Utah Agricultural Experiment Station.

References

1. Tomlinson B, Henderson G. Some quantitative cerebral findings in normal and demented old people. In: Terry RDGS, ed. Neurobiology of Aging. New York: Raven Press, 1976.

2. Glenner G. Congophilic microangiopathy in the pathogenesis of Alzheimer's syndrome (presenile dementia). Med Hypotheses 1979; 5:1231–1236.

3. Vinters H. Cerebral amyloid angiopathy: a critical review. Stroke 1987; 18:311–324.

4. Kalaria R, Hedera P. β-Amyloid vasoactivity in Alzheimer's disease [letter]. Lancet 1996; 347:1492–1493.

5. Perlmutter L, Chui HC. Micro-angiopathy, the vascular basement membrane and Alzheimer's disease: a review. Brain Res Bull 1990; 24:677–686.

6. Kimura T, Hashimura T, Miyakawa T. Observations of microvessels in the brain with Alzheimer's disease by scanning electron microscopy. Jpn Psychiatry Neurol 1991; 45:671–676.

7. Scheibel A, Duong T, Tomiyasu U. Denervation microangiopathy in senile dementia, Alzheimer type. Alzheimer Dis Assoc Disord 1987; 1:19–37.

8. Claudio L. Utrastructural features of the blood–brain barrier in biopsy tissue from Alzheimer's disease patients. Acta Neuropathol 1996; 91:6–14.

9. White L, Petrovich H, Hardman J et al. Cerebrovascular pathology and dementia in autopsied Honolulu–Asia Aging Study participants. Ann N Y Acad Sci 2002; 977:9–23.

10. Snowdon D, Greiner L, Mortimer J et al. Brain infarction and the clinical expression of Alzheimer disease. The Nun Study. JAMA 1997; 277:813–817.

11. Neuropathology Group. Medical Research Council Cognitive Function and Aging Study. Pathological correlates of late-onset dementia in a multicentre, community-based population in England and Wales. Neuropathology Group of the Medical Research Council Cognitive Function and Ageing Study (MRC CFAS). Lancet 2001; 357: 169–175.

12. Lim A, Tsuang D, Kukull W et al. Clinico-neuropathologic correlation of Alzheimer's disease in a commu-nity-based case series. J Am Geriatr Soc 1999; 47:564–569.

13. Nagy Z, Esiri M, Jobst K et al. The effects of additional pathology on the cognitive deficit in Alzheimer disease. J Neuropathol Exp Neurol 1997; 56:165–170.

14. Heyman A, Fillenbaum G, Welsh-Bohmer K et al. Cerebral infarcts in patients with autopsy-proven Alzheimer's disease: CERAD, part XVIII. Consortium to Establish a Registry for Alzheimer's Disease. Neurology 1998; 51:159–162.

15. Holmes C, Cairns N, Lantos P, Mann A. Validity of current clinical criteria for Alzheimer's disease, vascular dementia and dementia with Lewy bodies. Br J Psychiatry 1999; 174:45–50.

16. Davies L, Wolska B, Hilbich C et al. A4 amyloid protein deposition and the diagnosis of Alzheimer's disease: prevalence in aged brains determined by immunocytochemistry compared with conventional neuropathologic techniques. Neurology 1988; 38:1688–1693.

17. Delaère P, He Y, Fayet G et al. Beta A4 deposits are constant in the brain of the oldest old: an immuno-cytochemical study of 20 French centenarians. Neurobiol Aging 1993; 14:191–194.

18. Davis D, Schmitt F, Wekstein D, Markesbery W. Alzheimer neuropathologic alterations in aged cognitively normal subjects. J Neuropathol Exp Neurol 1999; 58:376–388.

19. Etiene D, Kraft J, Ganju N et al. Cerebrovascular pathology contributes to the heterogeneity of Alzheimer's disease. J Alzheimer Dis 1998; 1:119–134.

20. Erkinjuntti T, Hachinski V. Dementia post stroke. In: Teasell R, ed. Physical Medicine and Rehabilitation: State of the Art Reviews. Vol 7. Philadelphia: Hanley & Belfus, 1993:195–212.

21. Skoog I. A review on blood pressure and ischaemic white matter lesions. Dement Geriatr Cogn Disord 1998; 9(Suppl 1):13–19.

22. Blennow K, Wallin A, Uhlemann C, Gottfries C. White-matter lesions on CT in Alzheimer patients: relation to clinical symptomatology and vascular factors. Acta Neurol Scand 1991; 83:187–193.

23. Lotz P, Ballinger W Jr, Quisling R. Subcortical arteriosclerotic encephalopathy: CT spectrum and pathologic correlation. Am J Neuroradiol 1986; 7:817–822.

24. Brun A, Englund E. A white matter disorder in dementia of the Alzheimer type: a pathoanatomical study. Ann Neurol 1986; 19:253–262.

25. Scheltens P, Barkhof F, Valk J et al. White matter lesions on magnetic resonance imaging in clinically diagnosed Alzheimer's disease. Evidence for a heterogeneity. Brain 1992; 115:735–748.

26. Skoog I, Palmertz B, Andreasson LA. The prevalence of white-matter lesions on computed tomography of the brain in demented and nondemented 85-year-olds. J Geriatr Psychiatry Neurol 1994; 7:169–175.

27. Ogata J. Vascular dementia: the role of changes in the vessels. Alzheimer Dis Assoc Disord 1999; 13 Suppl 3:S55–58.

28. De la Monte S. Quantitation of cerebral atrophy in preclinical and end-stage Alzheimer's disease. Ann Neurol 1989; 25:450–459.

29. Skoog I, Lernfelt B, Landahl S et al. 15-year longitudinal study of blood pressure and dementia. Lancet 1996; 347:1141–1145.

30. Román G. Senile dementia of the Binswanger type. A vascular form of dementia in the elderly. JAMA 1987; 258:1782–1788.

31. Longstreth W, Manolio T, Arnold A et al. Clinical correlates of white matter findings on cranial magnetic resonance imaging of 3301 elderly people. The Cardiovascular Health Study. Stroke 1996; 27:1274–1282.

32. Schmidt R, Fazekas F, Koch M et al. Magnetic resonance imaging cerebral abnormalities and neuropsychological test performance in elderly hypertensive subjects. A case–control study. Arch Neurol 1995; 52:905–910.

33. de Leeuw FE, de Groot JC, Oudkerk M et al. Hypertension and cerebral white matter lesions in a prospective cohort study. Brain 2002; 125(Pt 4):765–772.

34. Skoog I, Wallin A, Fredman P et al. A population study on blood–brain barrier function in 85-year-olds: relation to Alzheimer's disease and vascular dementia. Neurology 1998; 50:966–971.

35. de la Torre J. Cerebral hypoperfusion, capillary degeneration, and development of Alzheimer disease. Alzheimer Dis Assoc Disord 2000; 14 (Suppl 1):S72–S81.

36. McKhann G, Drachman D, Folstein M et al. Clinical diagnosis of Alzheimer's disease: report of the NINCDS–ADRDA work group under the auspices of Department of Health and Human Services task

force on Alzheimer's disease. Neurology 1984; 34:939–944.

37. Vermeer SE, Prins ND, den Heijer T et al. Silent brain infarcts and the risk of dementia and cognitive decline. N Engl J Med 2003; 348:1215–1222.

38. Tatemichi TK, Paik M, Bagiella E et al. Risk of dementia after stroke in a hospitalized cohort: results of a longitudinal study. Neurology 1994; 44:1885–1891.

39. Skoog I. Status of risk factors for vascular dementia. Neuroepidemiology 1998; 17:2–9.

40. Skoog I. Vascular aspects in Alzheimer's disease. J Neural Transm Suppl 2000; 59:37–43.

41. Skoog I, Nilsson L, Palmertz B et al. A population-based study of dementia in 85-year-olds. N Engl J Med 1993; 328:153–158.

42. Skoog I. Risk factors for vascular dementia: a review. Dementia 1994; 5:137–144.

43. Chui H, Gonthier R. Natural history of vascular dementia. Alzheimer Dis Assoc Disord 1999; 13 Suppl 3:S124–130.

44. American Psychiatric Association. Diagnostic and Statistical Manual of Mental Disorders. 4th edn. Washington, DC, 1994.

45. Fischer P, Gatterer G, Marterer A et al. Course characteristics in the differentiation of dementia of the Alzheimer type and multi-infarct dementia. Acta Psychiatr Scand 1990; 81:551–553.

46. Skoog I, Vanmechelen E, Andreasson LA et al. A population-based study of tau protein and ubiquitin in cerebrospinal fluid in 85-year-olds: relation to severity of dementia and cerebral atrophy, but not to the apolipoprotein E4 allele. Neurodegeneration 1995; 4:433–442.

47. Skoog I, Davidsson P, Aevarsson O et al. Cerebrospinal fluid beta-amyloid 42 is reduced before the onset of sporadic dementia: a population-based study in 85-year-olds. Dement Geriatr Cogn Disord 2003; 15:169–176.

48. Sjögren M, Gustafson L, Wikkelso C, Wallin A. Frontotemporal dementia can be distinguished from Alzheimer's disease and subcortical white matter dementia by an anterior to posterior rCBF-SPET ratio. Dementia Geriatr Cogn Dis 2000; 11:275–285.

49. Vermeer SE, Den Heijer T, Koudstaal PJ et al. Incidence and risk factors of silent brain infarcts in the population-based Rotterdam Scan Study. Stroke 2003; 34:392–396.

50. Pasquier F, Leys D. Why are stroke patients prone to develop dementia? J Neurol 1997; 244:135–142.

51. Wetterling T, Kanitz R-D, Borgis K-J. Comparison of different diagnostic criteria for vascular dementia (ADDTC, DSM-IV, ICD-10, NINDS–AIREN). Stroke 1996; 27:30–36.

52. Amar K, Wilcock G, Scott M. The diagnosis of vascular dementia in the light of the new criteria. Age Ageing 1996; 25:51–55.

53. Ferrucci L, Guralnik J, Salive M et al. Cognitive impairment and risk of stroke in the older population. J Am Geriatr Soc 1996; 44:237–241.

54. Gale C, Martyn C, Cooper C. Cognitive impairment and mortality in a cohort of elderly people. BMJ 1996; 312:608–611.

55. Zhu L, Fratiglioni L, Guo Z et al. Incidence of stroke in relation to cognitive function and dementia in the Kungsholmen Project. Neurology 2000; 54:2103–2107.

56. Eastwood R, Amaducci L, Brayne C et al. The challenge of the dementias. Lancet 1996; 347:1303–1307.

57. Launer LJ, Ross GW, Petrovitch H, et al. Midlife blood pressure and dementia: the Honolulu–Asia Aging Study. Neurobiol Aging 2000; 21:49–55.

58. Kivipelto M, Helkala E-L, Laakso M et al. Midlife vascular risk factors and Alzheimer's disease in later life: longitudinal, population-based study. BMJ 2001; 322:1447–1451.

59. Kivipelto M, Helkala EL, Laakso MP et al. Apolipoprotein E epsilon4 allele, elevated midlife total cholesterol level, and high midlife systolic blood pressure are independent risk factors for late-life Alzheimer disease. Ann Intern Med 2002; 137:149–155.

60. Gustafson D, Rothenberg E, Blennow K et al. An 18-year follow-up of overweight and risk for Alzheimer's Disease. Arch Internal Med 2003; 163:1524–8.

61. Launer LJ. Demonstrating the case that AD is a vascular disease: epidemiologic evidence. Ageing Res Rev 2002; 1:61–77.

62. Ott A, Stolk RP, van Harskamp F et al. Diabetes mellitus and the risk of dementia: the Rotterdam Study. Neurology 1999; 53:1937–1942.

63. Skoog I. The interaction between vascular disorders and Alzheimer's disease. In: Wisniewski H, ed. Alzheimer's Disease and Related Disorders: Etiology, Pathogenesis and Therapeutics. Chichester:

John Wiley & Sons, 1999: 523–530.

64. Skoog I, Kalaria RN, Breteler MM. Vascular factors and Alzheimer disease. Alzheimer Dis Assoc Disord 1999; 13(Suppl 3):S106–114.

65. Kannel WB. Risk stratification in hypertension: new insights from the Framingham Study. Am J Hypertens 2000; 13(1 Pt 2):3S–10S.

66. Kalmijn S, Foley D, White L et al. Metabolic cardiovascular syndrome and risk of dementia in Japanese-American elderly men: the Honolulu–Asia aging study. Arterioscler Thromb Vasc Biol 2000; 20:2255–2260.

67. Kuusisto J, Koivisto K, Mykkanen L et al. Association between features of the insulin resistance syndrome and Alzheimer's disease independently of apolipoprotein E4 phenotype: cross-sectional population-based study. BMJ 1997; 315:1045–1049.

68. Dannenberg A, Garrison RJ, Kannell WB. Incidence of hypertension in the Framingham Study. Am J Publ Health 1988; 78:676–679.

69. Petrovitch H, White LR, Izmirilian G et al. Midlife blood pressure and neuritic plaques, neurofibrillary tangles, and brain weight at death: the HAAS. Honolulu–Asia Aging Study. Neurobiol Aging 2000; 21:57–62.

70. Sparks DL, Scheff SW, Liu H et al. Increased incidence of neurofibrillary tangles (NFT) in non-demented individuals with hypertension. J Neurol Sci 1995; 131:162–169.

71. Qiu C, von Strauss E, Fastbom J et al. Low blood pressure and risk of dementia in the Kungsholmen project: a 6-year follow-up study. Arch Neurol 2003; 60:223–228.

72. Ruitenberg A. Vascular Factors in Dementia. Observations in the Rotterdam Study. Rotterdam: Erasmus University, 2000.

73. Wu C, Zhou D, Wen C et al. Relationship between blood pressure and Alzheimer's disease in Linxian County, China. Life Sci 2003; 72:1125–1133.

74. Posner HB, Tang MX, Luchsinger J et al. The relationship of hypertension in the elderly to AD, vascular dementia, and cognitive function. Neurology 2002; 58:1175–1181.

75. Yoshitake T, Kiyohara Y, Kato I et al. Incidence and risk factors of vascular dementia and Alzheimer's disease in a defined elderly Japanese population: the Hisayama Study. Neurology 1995; 45:1161–1168.

76. Morris MC, Scherr PA, Hebert LE et al. Association of incident Alzheimer disease and blood pressure measured from 13 years before to 2 years after diagnosis in a large community study. Arch Neurol 2001; 58:1640–1646.

77. Yamada M, Kasagi F, Sasaki H et al. Association between dementia and midlife risk factors: the Radiation Effects Research Foundation Adult Health Study. J Am Geriatr Soc 2003; 51:410–414.

78. Qiu C, Winblad B, Viitanen M, Fratiglioni L. Pulse pressure and risk of Alzheimer disease in persons aged 75 years and older: a community-based, longitudinal study. Stroke 2003; 34:594–599.

79. Murray CJ, Lauer JA, Hutubessy RC et al. Effectiveness and costs of interventions to lower systolic blood pressure and cholesterol: a global and regional analysis on reduction of cardiovascular-disease risk. Lancet 2003; 361:717–725.

80. Guo Z, Viitanen M, Fratiglioni L, Winblad B. Low blood pressure and dementia in elderly people: the Kungsholmen project. BMJ 1996; 312:805–808.

81. Skoog I, Andreasson LA, Landahl S, Lernfelt B. A population-based study on blood pressure and brain atrophy in 85-year-olds. Hypertension 1998; 32:404–409.

82. Hogan D, Ebly E, Rockwood K. Weight, blood pressure, osmolarity, and glucose levels across various stages of Alzheimer's disease and vascular dementia. Dement Geriatr Cogn Disord 1997; 8:147–151.

83. Ruitenberg A, Skoog I, Ott A et al. Blood pressure and risk of dementia: results from the Rotterdam Study and the Gothenburg H-70 Study. Dement Geriatr Cogn Disord 2001; 12:33–39.

84. Guo Z, Viitanen M, Winblad B, Fratiglioni L. Low blood pressure and incidence of dementia in a very old sample: dependent on initial cognition. J Am Geriatr Soc 1999; 47:723–726.

85. Burke W, Coronado P, Schmitt C et al. Blood pressure regulation in Alzheimer's disease. J Auton Nerv Syst 1994; 48:65–71.

86. Passant U. Posture and brain function in dementia. A study with special reference to orthostatic hypotension. Thesis. University of Lund, 1996.

87. Chalmer J, Arnolda L, Smith I et al. Central nervous control of blood pressure. In: Swales J, ed. Textbook of Hypertension. Oxford: Blackwell Scientific, 1994; 409–426.

88. Reis D. The brain and hypertension. Arch Neurol 1988; 45:180–183.

89. Lantos P, Cairns N. The neuropathology of Alzheimer's disease. In: Levy R, ed. Dementia. London: Chapman and Hall, 1994: 185–207.

90. Adams J, Brierley J, Connor R, Treip C. The effects of systemic hypotension upon the human brain. Clinical and neuropathologic observations in 11 cases. Brain 1966; 89:235–267.

91. Guo Z, Fratiglioni L, Zhu L et al. Occurrence and progression of dementia in a community population aged 75 years and older: relationship of antihypertensive medication use. Arch Neurol 1999; 56:991–996.

92. Guo Z, Fratiglioni L, Viitanen M et al. Apolipoprotein E genotypes and the incidence of Alzheimer's disease among persons aged 75 years and older: variation by use of antihypertensive medication? Am J Epidemiol 2001; 153:225–231.

93. Richards SS, Emsley CL, Roberts J et al. The association between vascular risk factor-mediating medications and cognition and dementia diagnosis in a community-based sample of African-Americans. J Am Geriatr Soc 2000; 48:1035–1041.

94. in't Veld BA, Ruitenberg A, Hofman A et al. Antihypertensive drugs and incidence of dementia: the Rotterdam Study. Neurobiol Aging 2001; 22:407–412.

95. Forette F, Seux M-L, Staessen J et al. Prevention of dementia in randomised double-blind placebo-controlled Systolic Hypertension in Europe (Syst-Eur) trial. Lancet 1998; 352:1347–1351.

96. Forette F, Seux ML, Staessen JA et al. The prevention of dementia with antihypertensive treatment: new evidence from the Systolic Hypertension in Europe (Syst-Eur) study. Arch Intern Med 2002; 162:2046–2052.

97. Prince MJ, Bird AS, Blizard RA, Mann AH. Is the cognitive function of older patients affected by antihypertensive treatment? Results from 54 months of the Medical Research Council's trial of hypertension in older adults. BMJ 1996; 312:801–805.

98. Lithell H, Hansson L, Skoog I et al. The Study on COgnition and Prognosis in the Elderly (SCOPE). Principal results of a randomised double-blind intervention trial. J Hypertens 2003; 21:875–886.

99. van Bockxmeer F, Mamotte C. Apolipoprotein E4 homozygosity in young men with coronary heart disease. Lancet 1992; 340:879–880.

100. Wilson P, Myers R, Larson M et al. Apolipoprotein E alleles, dyslipidemia, and coronary heart disease: the Framingham offspring study. JAMA 1994; 272:1666–1671.

101. Davignon J, Gregg R, Sing C. Apolipoprotein E polymorphism and atherosclerosis. Arteriosclerosis 1988; 8:1–21.

102. Eto M, Watanabe K, Chonan N, Ishii K. Familial hypercholesterolemia and apolipoprotein E4. Atherosclerosis 1988; 72: 123–128.

103. Polvikoski T, Sulkava R, Haltia M et al. Apolipoprotein E, dementia, and cortical deposition of β-amyloid protein. N Engl J Med 1995; 333:1242–1247.

104. Corder E, Saunders A, Strittmatter W et al. Gene dose of apolipoprotein E type 4 allele and the risk of Alzheimer's disease in late onset families. Science 1993; 261:921–923.

105. Poirier J, Davignon J, Bouthillier D et al. Apolipoprotein E polymorphism and Alzheimer's disease. Lancet 1993; 342:697–699.

106. Saunders A, Strittmatter W, Schmechel D et al. Association of apolipoprotein E allele e4 with late-onset familial and sporadic Alzheimer's disease. Neurology 1993; 43:1467–1472.

107. Hofman A, Ott A, Breteler MM et al. Atherosclerosis, apolipoprotein E, and prevalence of dementia and Alzheimer's disease in the Rotterdam Study. Lancet 1997; 349:151–154.

108. Aevarsson O, Svanborg A, Skoog I. Seven-year survival rate after age 85 years: relation to Alzheimer disease and vascular dementia. Arch Neurol 1998; 55:1226–1232.

109. Mahley R. Apolipoprotein E: cholesterol transport protein with expanding role in cell biology. Science 1988; 240:622–630.

110. Mahley R. Heparan sulfate proteoglycan/low density lipoprotein receptor-related protein pathway involved in type III hyperlipoproteinemia and Alzheimer's disease. Isr J Med Sci 1996; 32:414–429.

111. Davignon J, Bouthillier D, Nestruck A, Sing C. Apolipoprotein E polymorphism and atherosclerosis: insight from a study in octogenarians. Trans Am Clin Climatol Assoc 1987; 99:100–110.

112. Campbell J, Campbell G. Pathogenesis of atheroma. In: Swales J, ed. Textbook of Hypertension. Oxford: Blackwell Scientific, 1994.

113. Bales KR, Verina T, Dodel RC et al. Lack of apolipoprotein E dramatically reduces amyloid beta-peptide deposition. Nat Genet 1997; 17:263–264.

114. Brendza RP, Bales KR, Paul SM, Holtzman DM. Role of apoE/Abeta interactions in Alzheimer's disease: insights from transgenic mouse models. Mol Psychiatry 2002; 7:132–135.

115. Launer LJ, White LR, Petrovitch H et al. Cholesterol and neuropathologic markers of AD. A population-based autopsy study. Neurology 2001; 57:1447–1452.

116. Sparks D. Coronary artery disease, hypertension, ApoE, and cholesterol: a link to Alzheimer's disease? Ann N Y Acad Sci 1997; 826:128–146.

117. Notkola I-L, Sulkava R, Pekkanen J et al. Serum total cholesterol, apolipoprotein E e4 allele, and Alzheimer's disease. Neuroepidemiology 1998; 17:14–20.

118. Sparks DL, Liu H, Gross DR, Scheff SW. Increased density of cortical apolipoprotein E immunoreactive neurons in rabbit brain after dietary administration of cholesterol. Neurosci Lett 1995; 187:142–144.

119. Simons M, Keller P, De Strooper B et al. Cholesterol depletion inhibits the generation of beta-amyloid in hippocampal neurons. Proc Natl Acad Sci USA 1998; 95:6460–6464.

120. Fassbender K, Simons M, Bergmann C et al. Simvastatin strongly reduces levels of Alzheimer's disease beta-amyloid

peptides Abeta 42 and Abeta 40 in vitro and in vivo. Proc Natl Acad Sci USA 2001; 10:10.

121. Refolo LM, Malester B, LaFrancois J et al. Hypercholesterolemia accelerates the Alzheimer's amyloid pathology in a transgenic mouse model. Neurobiol Dis 2000; 7:321–331.

122. Refolo LM, Pappolla MA, LaFrancois J et al. A cholesterol-lowering drug reduces beta-amyloid pathology in a transgenic mouse model of Alzheimer's disease. Neurobiol Dis 2001; 8:890–899.

123. Jick H, Zornberg GL, Jick SS et al. Statins and the risk of dementia. Lancet 2000; 356: 1627–1631.

124. Wolozin B, Kellman W, Ruosseau P et al. Decreased prevalence of Alzheimer disease associated with 3-hydroxy-3-methyglutaryl coenzyme A reductase inhibitors. Arch Neurol 2000; 57:1439–1443.

125. Rockwood K, Kirkland S, Hogan DB et al. Use of lipid-lowering agents, indication bias, and the risk of dementia in community-dwelling elderly people. Arch Neurol 2002; 59:223–227.

126. Simons M, Schwarzler F, Lutjohann D et al. Treatment with simvastatin in normocholesterolemic patients with Alzheimer's disease: a 26-week randomized, placebo-controlled, double-blind trial. Ann Neurol 2002; 52:346–350.

127. Sjögren M, Gustafsson K, Syversen S et al. Treatment with simvastatin in patients with Alzheimer's disease lowers both alpha- and beta-cleaved APP. Dement Geriatr Cogn Dis 2003; 16:25–30.

128. Peila R, Rodriguez BL, Launer LJ. Type 2 diabetes, APOE gene, and the risk for dementia and related pathologies: the Honolulu–Asia Aging Study. Diabetes 2002; 51:1256–1262.

129. Leibson C, Rocca W, Hanson V et al. Risk of dementia among persons with diabetes mellitus: a population-based cohort study. Am J Epidemiol 1997; 145:301–308.

130. Curb J, Rodriguez B, Abbott R et al. Longitudinal association of vascular and Alzheimer's dementias, diabetes, and glucose tolerance. Neurology 1999; 52:971–975.

131. MacKnight C, Rockwood K, Awalt E, McDowell I. Diabetes mellitus and the risk of dementia, Alzheimer's disease and vascular cognitive impairment in the Canadian Study of Health and Aging. Dement Geriatr Cogn Disord 2002; 14:77–83.

132. Hassing LB, Johansson B, Nilsson SE et al. Diabetes mellitus is a risk factor for vascular dementia, but not for Alzheimer's disease: a population-based study of the oldest old. Int Psychogeriatr 2002; 14:239–248.

133. Mooradian AD. Central nervous system complications of diabetes mellitus—a perspective from the blood–brain barrier. Brain Res Brain Res Rev 1997; 23:210–218.

134. Singh R, Barden A, Mori T, Beilin L. Advanced glycation end-products: a review. Diabetologia 2001; 44:129–146.

135. Stern DM, Yan SD, Yan SF, Schmidt AM. Receptor for advanced glycation endproducts (RAGE) and the complications of

diabetes. Ageing Res Rev 2002; 1:1–15.

136. Yan S, Chen X, Fu J et al. RAGE and amyloid-β peptide neurotoxicity in Alzheimer's disease. Nature 1996; 382:685–691.

137. Vitek MP, Bhattacharya K, Glendening JM et al. Advanced glycation end products contribute to amyloidosis in Alzheimer disease. Proc Natl Acad Sci USA 1994; 91:4766–4770.

138. Gasparini L, Netzer W, Greengard P, Xu H. Does insulin dysfunction play a role in Alzheimer's disease? Trends Pharmacol Sci 2002; 23:288–293.

139. Mooradian AD. Pathophysiology of central nervous system complications in diabetes mellitus. Clin Neurosci 1997; 4:322–326.

140. Aronson M, Ooi W, Morgenstern H et al. Women, myocardial infarction, and dementia in the very old. Neurology 1990; 40:1102–1106.

141. Soneira C, Scott T. Severe cardiovascular disease and Alzheimer's disease: senile plaque formation in cortical areas. Clin Anat 1996; 9:118–127.

142. Sparks D, Hunsaker J III, Scheff S et al. Cortical senile plaques in coronary artery disease, aging and Alzheimer's disease. Neurobiol Aging 1990; 11:601–607.

143. Ott A, Breteler MM, de Bruyne MC et al. Atrial fibrillation and dementia in a population-based study. The Rotterdam Study. Stroke 1997; 28:316–321.

144. de Leeuw FE, de Groot JC, Oudkerk M et al. Atrial fibrillation and the risk of cerebral white matter lesions. Neurology 2000; 54:1795–1801.

145. Zito M, Muscari A, Marini E et al. Silent lacunar infarcts in elderly patients with chronic nonvalvular atrial fibrillation. Aging (Milano) 1996; 8:341–346.

146. de Leeuw FE, de Groot JC, Bots ML et al. Carotid atherosclerosis and cerebral white matter lesions in a population-based magnetic resonance imaging study. J Neurol 2000; 247:291–296.

147. Lethem R, Orrell M. Antioxidants and dementia. Lancet 1997; 349:1189–1190.

148. El Khoury J, Hickman S, Thomas C et al. Scavenger receptor-mediated adhesion of microglia to β-amyloid fibrils. Nature 1996; 382:716–719.

149. Thomas T, Thomas G, McLendon C et al. β-Amyloid-mediated vasoactivity and vascular endothelial damage. Nature 1996; 380:168–171.

150. Finkel E. Pinning the suspect to the crime in Alzheimer's. Lancet 1996; 348:1506.

151. Sinclair A, Bayer A, Johnston J et al. Altered plasma antioxidant status in subjects with Alzheimer's disease and vascular dementia. Int J Geriatr Psychiatry 1998; 13:840–845.

152. Jendroska K, Poewe W, Daniel S et al. Ischemic stress induces deposition of amyloid β immunoreactivity in human brain. Acta Neuropathol 1995; 90:461–466.

153. Hall E, Oostveen J, Dunn E, Carter D. Increased amyloid protein precursor and apolipoprotein E immunoreactivity in the selectively

vulnerable hippocampus following transient forebrain ischemia in gerbils. Exp Neurol 1995; 135:17–27.

154. Bennett SA, Pappas BA, Stevens WD et al. Cleavage of amyloid precursor protein elicited by chronic cerebral hypoperfusion. Neurobiol Aging 2000; 21:207–214.

155. Kalaria R, Bhatti S, Palatinsky E et al. Accumulation of the beta amyloid precursor protein at sites of ischemic injury in rat brain. Neuroreport 1993; 4:211–214.

156. Stephenson DT, Rash K, Clemens JA. Amyloid precursor protein accumulates in regions of neurodegeneration following focal cerebral ischemia in the rat. Brain Res 1992; 593:128–135.

157. Pennypacker K, Hernandez H, Benkovic S et al. Induction of presenilins in the rat brain after middle cerebral arterial occlusion. Brain Res Bull 1999; 48:539–543.

158. Tanimukai H, Imaizumi K, Kudo T et al. Alzheimer-associated presenilin-1 gene is induced in gerbil hippocampus after transient ischemia. Brain Res Mol Brain Res 1998; 54:212–218.

159. Citron M, Eckman C, Diehl T et al. Additive effects of PS1 and APP mutations on secretion of the 42-residue amyloid beta-protein. Neurobiol Dis 1998; 5:107–116.

160. Sudoh S, Kawamura Y, Sato S et al. Presenilin 1 mutations linked to familial Alzheimer's disease increase the intracellular levels of amyloid beta-protein 1-42 and its N-terminally truncated variant(s) which are generated at distinct sites. J Neurochem 1998; 71:1535–1543.

161. Henderson A. The risk factors for Alzheimer's disease: a review and a hypothesis. Acta Psychiatr Scand 1988; 78:257–275.

162. Ghribi O, Lapierre L, Girard M et al. Hypoxia-induced loss of synaptic transmission is exacerbated in hippocampal slices of transgenic mice expressing C-terminal fragments of Alzheimer amyloid precursor protein. Hippocampus 1999; 9:201–205.

163. Mooradian A. Effect of aging on the blood–brain barrier. Neurobiol Aging 1988; 9:31–39.

164. Johansson B. Cerebral vascular bed in hypertension and consequences for the brain. Hypertension 1984; 6 (Suppl 3):81–86.

165. Johansson B. Pathogenesis of vascular dementia: the possible role of hypertension. Dementia 1994; 5:174–176.

166. Nag S. Cerebral changes in chronic hypertension: combined permeability and immunohistochemical studies. Acta Neuropathol (Berl) 1984; 62:178–184.

167. Shah GN, Mooradian AD. Age-related changes in the blood–brain barrier. Exp Gerontol 1997; 32:501–519.

168. Hardy J, Mann D, Wester P, Winblad B. An integrative hypothesis concerning the pathogenesis and progression of Alzheimer's disease. Neurobiol Aging 1986; 7:489–502.

169. Kalaria R, Golde T, Cohen M, Younkin S. Serum amyloid P in Alzheimer's disease. Implications for dysfunction of the blood–brain barrier. Ann N Y Acad Sci 1991; 640:145–148.

170. Perlmutter L, Myers M, Barrón E. Vascular basement membrane components and the lesions of Alzheimer's disease: light and electron microscopic analyses. Micros Res Tech 1994; 28:204–215.

171. Hampel H, Muller-Spahn F, Berger C et al. Evidence of blood–cerebrospinal fluid-barrier impairment in a subgroup of patients with dementia of the Alzheimer type and major depression: a possible indicator for immunoactivation. Dementia 1995; 6:348–354.

172. Elovaara I, Seppälä I, Palo J et al. Oligo-clonal immunoglobulin bands in cerebrospinal fluid of patients with Alzheimer's disease and vascular dementia. Acta Neurol Scand 1988; 77:397–401.

173. Blennow K, Wallin A, Fredman P et al. Blood–brain barrier disturbance in patients with Alzheimer's disease is related to vascular factors. Acta Neurol Scand 1990; 81:349–351.

174. Mecocci P, Parnetti L, Reboldi G et al. Blood–brain barrier in a geriatric population: barrier function in degenerative and vascular dementia. Acta Neurol Scand 1991; 84:210–213.

175. Kay A, May C, Papadopoulos N et al. CSF and serum concentration of albumin and IgG in Alzheimer's disease. Neurobiol Aging 1987; 8:21–25.

176. Leonardi A, Gandolfo C, Caponetto C et al. The integrity of the blood–brain barrier in Alzheimer's type and multi-infarct dementia evaluated by the study of albumin and IgG in serum and cerebrospinal fluid. J Neurol Sci 1985; 67:253–261.

177. Bader M, Paul M, Fernandez-Alfonso M et al. Molecular biology and biochemistry of the renin–angiotensin system. In: Swales J, ed. Textbook of Hypertension. Oxford: Blackwell Scientific, 1994.

178. Struijker Boudier H. Vascular growth and hypertension. In: Swales J, ed. Textbook of Hypertension. Oxford: Blackwell Scientific, 1994.

179. Baumbach G, Heistad D. Cerebrovascular disease in experimental models of hypertension. In: Swales J, ed. Textbook of Hypertension. Oxford: Blackwell Scientific, 1994.

180. Schiffrin E, Deng L, Larochelle P. Progressive improvement in the structure of resistance arteries of hypertensive patients after 2 years of treatment with an angiotensin I-converting enzyme inhibitor. Comparison with effects of a β-blocker. J Hypertens 1995; 8:229–236.

181. Wright J, Harding J. Brain angiotensin receptor subtypes in the control of physiological and behavioral responses. Neurosci Biobehav R 1994; 18:21–53.

182. Barnes J, Barnes N, Costall B et al. Angiotensin II inhibits the release of [3H]acetylcholine from rat entorhinal cortex in vitro. Brain Res 1989; 492:136–143.

183. Barnes N, Champaneria S, Costall B et al. Cognitive enhancing actions of DUP 753 detected in a mouse habituation paradigm. Neuroreport 1990; 1:239–242.

184. Arregui A, Perry E, Rossor M, Tomlinson B. Angiotensin converting enzyme in Alzheimer's disease: increased activity in

caudate nucleus and cortical areas. J Neurochem 1982; 82:1490–1492.

185. Barnes N, Cheng C, Costall B et al. Angiotensin converting enzyme density is increased in temporal cortex from patients with Alzheimer's disease. Eur J Pharmacol 1991; 20:289–292.

186. Ekeberg O, Kjeldsen S, Eide I, Leren P. Childhood traumas and psychosocial characteristics of 50-year-old men with essential hypertension. J Psychosom Res 1990; 34:643–649.

187. Persson G, Skoog I. A prospective population study of psychosocial risk factors for late-onset dementia. Int J Geriatric Psychiatry 1996; 11:15–22.

188. Meaney M, Aitken D, van Berkel C et al. Effect of neonatal handling on age-related impairments associated with the hippocampus. Science 1988; 239:766–768.

189. Sapolsky R, Armanini M, Packan D, Tombaugh G. Stress and glucocorticoids in aging. Endocrinol Metabol Clin N Am 1987; 16:965–980.

190. Skoog I, Gustafson D. HRT and dementia. J Epidemiol Biostat 1999; 4:227–251; discussion 252.

191. Orgogozo JM, Dartigues JF, Lafont S et al. Wine consumption and dementia in the elderly: a prospective community study in the Bordeaux area. Rev Neurol (Paris) 1997; 153:185–192.

192. Sano M, Ernesto C, Thomas R et al. A controlled trial of selegiline, alpha-tocopherol, or both as treatment for Alzheimer's disease. N Engl J Med 1997; 336:1216–1222.

193. van Duijn C, Hofman A. Relation between nicotine intake and Alzheimer's disease. BMJ 1991; 302:1491–1494.

194. Graves AB, van Duijn CM, Chandra V et al. Alcohol and tobacco consumption as risk factors for Alzheimer's disease: a collaborative reanalysis of case–control studies. EURODEM Risk Factors Research Group. Int J Epidemiol 1991; 20(Suppl 2):S48–57.

195. Ott A, Slooter AJ, Hofman A et al. Smoking and risk of dementia and Alzheimer's disease in a population-based cohort study: the Rotterdam Study. Lancet 1998; 351:1840–1843.

196. Launer LJ, Andersen K, Dewey ME et al. Rates and risk factors for dementia and Alzheimer's disease: results from EURODEM pooled analyses. EURODEM Incidence Research Group and Work Groups. European Studies of Dementia. Neurology 1999; 52:78–84.

197. Wang HX, Fratiglioni L, Frisoni GB et al. Smoking and the occurrence of Alzheimer's disease: cross-sectional and longitudinal data in a population-based study. Am J Epidemiol 1999; 149:640–644.

198. Fratiglioni L, Wang HX. Smoking and Parkinson's and Alzheimer's disease: review of the epidemiological studies. Behav Brain Res 2000; 113:117–120.

199. Luscher T. Local relaxant and constricting factors in the vessel wall. In: Swales J, editor. Textbook of Hypertension. Oxford: Blackwell Scientific, 1994.

200. Umans J. Less nitric oxide, more pressure, or the converse? Lancet 1997; 349:816.

201. Suo Z, Humphrey J, Kundtz A et al. Soluble Alzheimer's beta-amyloid constricts the cerebral vasculature in vivo. Neurosci Lett 1998; 257:77–80.

202. Su GC, Arendash GW, Kalaria RN et al. Intravascular infusions of soluble beta-amyloid compromise the blood–brain barrier, activate CNS glial cells and induce peripheral hemorrhage. Brain Res 1999; 818:105–117.

203. Arendash G, Su G, Crawford F et al. Intravascular beta-amyloid infusion increases blood pressure: implications for a vasoactive role of beta-amyloid in the pathogenesis of Alzheimer's disease. Neurosci Lett 1999; 268:17–20.

204. Erkinjuntti T, Kurz A, Gauthier S et al. Efficacy of galantamine in probable vascular dementia and Alzheimer's disease combined with cerebrovascular disease: a randomised trial. Lancet 2002; 359:1283–1290.

205. Skoog I. Possibilities for secondary prevention of Alzheimer's disease. In: Christen Y, ed. The Epidemiology of Alzheimer's Disease: From Gene to Prevention. Berlin: Springer Verlag, 1999; 121–134.

3
The role of white-matter lesions in dementia

Leonardo Pantoni

Introduction

The relationship between cerebral white-matter lesions (WML) and cognitive performance has been one of the most controversial issues since the first descriptions of these changes by neuroimaging techniques in the early 1980s. Some of the aspects of this complex interaction have been summarized in recent review papers or editorials.[1–4] In this chapter, I will focus on some of the most burning questions in the field:

1) Do WML cause or contribute to the occurrence of dementia?
2) What is the contribution of WML to specific types of mental impairment, such as Alzheimer's disease (AD) and vascular dementia (VaD)?
3) Is there a role for WML in mild cognitive impairment and in predicting dementia onset?
4) Can WML be considered a surrogate marker of a specific form of dementia or cognitive impairment?

Other important issues, such as the role of WML in nondemented subjects, are beyond the aim of this chapter and will therefore not be dealt with.

Do white-matter lesions cause or contribute to the occurrence of dementia?

Early studies conducted in the 1980s suggested that WML, at that time mostly detected by computed tomography (CT), could represent a marker of dementia. These studies have been reviewed in detail elsewhere.[1] Many of them suffered from methodological limitations but generally demonstrated a higher frequency of WML in demented patients than nondemented subjects; when more accurate analyses were performed, however, the role of confounding factors such as a history of stroke also emerged.[5]

A second group of studies tested the hypothesis that the presence of WML is associated with a more severe degree of dementia, but, again, the results were not consistent. Studies based on CT examination tended to reveal more severe cognitive deficits in demented patients if they also had

WML.[6–11] This trend was absent in magnetic resonance imaging (MRI) studies, the majority of which, probably due to the lower specificity of MRI than that of CT, failed to find associations between the presence of WML and cognitive test scores, in many cases represented by the Mini-Mental State Examination (MMSE).[12–27] These studies, however, suffered from a number of shortcomings. First, some of these reports were based on small samples of subjects. Second, in many instances, patients of different age groups and with heterogeneous diseases were included. Third, the cognitive measures used were not consistent across the studies.

The third point appears to be crucial. In most studies, the presence of WML tended to influence more the performance on tests exploring specific cognitive functions than global cognitive functions.[13] For example, Almkvist et al observed that demented patients with WML were more impaired in tests evaluating visuoconstruction, attention, and finger-motor speed than patients without WML, despite comparable scores on tests of global cognitive function.[22] This finding is quite consistent in the literature on WML, even when studies on nondemented patients are considered.[28–35] The cognitive performances affected are those related to the integrity of subcortical-frontal circuits whose connecting white-matter pathways are probably damaged by the presence of WML.

Fourth, many studies did not differentiate WML location and severity and did not take into account the weight of other possibly coexisting brain abnormalities, such as cortical atrophy.[36]

The possible contribution of WML to dementia has also been evaluated in an autopsy-based study performed with postmortem MRI of 52 brains of subjects participating in the Nun Study.[37] These authors found a correlation of dementia diagnosis with volume of white matter, but not with WML visual rating. No correlation was found between WML scores and neuropsychological test performances (MMSE, delayed word recall, naming, and verbal fluency) or instrumental daily activities.[37] However, it should be noted that the use of postmortem MRI makes these data difficult to compare with the already mentioned in vivo studies, and that most of the cognitive tests did not aim to evaluate subcortical dysfunction. Finally, it should be determined to what extent white-matter volume is influenced by the presence of WML.

What are the contributions of white-matter lesions in specific types of mental impairment such as Alzheimer's disease and vascular dementia?

A particular and relevant issue is that of the significance of WML in AD. AD is considered to be the prototypic form of cortical dementia, yet it has been demonstrated that a large number of patients with AD (up to more than 50%) also have pathologically detected WML.[38] The two main questions in this sense concern the cause of WML in AD and their clinical significance. As originally pointed out by Brun and Englund,[38] the histologic appearance of WML in AD resembles that of incomplete infarct; thus, WML have been considered to be of possible vascular origin also in AD.[39] Therefore, WML are considered to be one of the vascular features of AD.[40,41] However, the real nature of WML in AD remains to be further elucidated, and the type of vessel damage responsible for the ischemic damage may be disputed. Moreover, mechanisms other than ischemia (such as blood–brain barrier damage) have also been hypothesized as a possible cause of WML in AD.[39,42]

A number of studies have reported on the clinical significance of WML in AD. Harrell et al[19] showed poorer neuropsychological performance in AD patients with severe WML than in those with mild WML. Scheltens et al[43] reported that the severity of WML was highly correlated with the age of onset of AD, which was much more severe in patients with senile onset (after 65 years), suggesting a microvessel comorbidity in this age group. Fazekas et al[44] showed that their 30 AD patients had a greater volume of periventricular WML than normal controls, and that both periventricular WML and measures of brain atrophy were predictors of a diagnosis of AD; however, when the variables were studied in a multivariate model, only brain-atrophy measures remained a predictor of AD. A group of studies have observed the presence of WML in AD to be associated with subcortical clinical features. Bennett et al[23] found no difference in disease severity (as expressed by the MMSE score) between AD patients with and without WML. However, WML were associated with gait disturbances and urinary incontinence, and, thus, with possibly higher levels of disability.[23] Starkstein et al[27] observed that their 15 AD patients with WML were significantly more apathetic and had extrapyramidal signs significantly more often than the remaining 23 AD patients without WML. No major differences were seen on a broad neuropsychological battery.[27] These results have been recently corroborated and partly expanded by Hirono and coworkers.[45] In their 76 Japanese AD patients, WML severity was found to be significantly associated with urinary incontinence, grasp reflex, and aberrant motor behavior. However, no association could be demonstrated with cognitive tests, such as the MMSE, the Wechsler Adult Intelligence Scale, and the Alzheimer's Disease Assessment Scale, that are strongly influenced by brain atrophy.[45] In a group of 158 AD patients, Marder et al[24] tested whether the presence of periventricular WML could influence disease severity, as assessed by the modified MMSE and part I of the Blessed Dementia Rating Scale. They found no significant difference on these two tests, while patients with WML tended to have a higher ischemic score than those without WML, reinforcing the idea that these changes might represent expression of underlying vascular pathology.[24]

Another specific issue is the potential role of WML in the development of dementia after stroke. This question has been dealt with in a few studies performed in unselected stroke patient series[46–49] or lacunar stroke series;[50,51] with few exceptions,[49,51] WML were found to be a significant and independent risk factor for post-stroke dementia. In all these studies, including those with negative findings, the definition of dementia relied on the determination of cognitive deficits related more to cortical than to subcortical structure dysfunction. This might have even lessened the appreciation of the overall predictive value in WML in relation to cognitive impairment in stroke patients. The issue of post-stroke dementia is also complicated by the existence of patients who were demented before stroke. Interestingly, WML have also been found to be one of the factors associated with prestroke dementia.[52–54]

A position paper, published in 1999, devoted to the issue of the role of WML in vascular cognitive impairment,[55] reported that some forms of VaD are apparently sustained solely by the presence of WML, and suggested that WML per se can cause dementia in some instances. The cognitive impairment associated with the presence of WML is thought to be caused by the disruption of cortical-subcortical circuits.[56,57] However, the position paper also stated that the presence of WML is not synonymous with dementia, and outlined some of the obstacles in the clarification of the role of WML in cognitive impairment.[55] One of the many difficulties is probably the fact that WML are only one aspect of vascular brain changes in the elderly with potential and actual influence on cognitive performances. Possibly, there is a complex interaction between coexisting vascular lesions that represents the correlate of dementia. In this sense, WML are likely to be an indicator of, but not the only factor causing, dementia.

Is there a role for white-matter lesions in mild cognitive impairment and in predicting dementia onset?

Although not sufficient to explain the full dementia syndrome in most instances, the fact that WML of a certain severity are almost invariably associated with some degree of cognitive deficit, in particular of the frontal lobe type,[55] leads to the hypothesis that their presence causes mild cognitive impairment and is a predictor of poor cognitive outcome at follow-up. So far, data on this longitudinal aspect are scanty. A preliminary study to test possible radiologic markers of the transition from mild cognitive impairment to dementia found that CT-detected WML and temporal lobe atrophy were significant predictors of AD in a small group of 27 patients.[58] Very recently, data from a large population-based study enrolling over 700 subjects demonstrated that the presence of WML (together with that of silent lacunar infarcts) significantly predicts dementia onset.[59] The hazard ratio of becoming demented over a 3.6-year follow-up was about 1.6 for subjects with periventricular WML at baseline MRI.[59]

In recent years, the concept of 'cognitive impairment no dementia of vascular origin' has been developed.[60] The new attention to this issue has led to the recognition of many patients who cannot be diagnosed with dementia, but who cannot be considered completely normal.[61,62] The issue is of great interest because it is proposed that these patients are in a predementia state and that a considerable proportion of them will develop the full clinical picture over a certain period.[63,64] Therefore, strategies aimed at preventing dementia could be particularly suited for this group of patients. In this sense, radiologic markers of mild cognitive impairment could help in detecting such cases and also in identifying possible subgroups at different risks of dementia. WML are among the lesions likely to be found associated with vascular cognitive impairment without dementia.[55] This has been substantiated by recent observations. Koga et al[65] examined a Japanese population sample of 254 subjects aged 60–91 years, nondemented and independent in activities of daily living, and defined 46 of them as mildly cognitively impaired, on the basis of a MMSE score of < 24 and the lack of fulfillment of the DSM-IV criteria for dementia. In this group, a quantitative MRI assessment of brain changes showed larger quantities of WML to be one of the significant factors predicting cognitive impairment in the multivariate analysis, together with cerebral atrophy and lower education level. In the National Heart, Lung, and Blood Institute Twin Study, WML volume, together with increasing age, apoliproprotein E4 genotype, elevated midlife blood pressure, and lower alcohol consumption, increased the risk of mild cognitive impairment in the multivariate analysis.[66] Subjects defined as affected by mild cognitive impairment had double volumes of WML in respect of controls (0.56% of cranial volume versus 0.25%).[66]

Can white-matter lesions be considered a surrogate marker of a specific form of dementia or cognitive impairment?

The possibility that WML, detected by either MRI or CT, could help in the differential diagnosis between VaD and AD had already been suggested in 1987.[67] Although the frequency of WML is generally higher in VaD than in AD,[68] the mere presence of these changes cannot be considered an unquestionable marker of any specific form of dementia. However, when not only the presence but also the extension of WML is taken into account, things may be different. In fact, in recent years, neuroimaging has become, together with a detailed analysis of the cognitive and behavioral syndrome, essential in the diagnosis of VaD.[64] The NINDS–AIREN criteria have proposed that extensive WML are one of the radiologic hallmarks of VaD. These criteria have arbitrarily chosen a cutoff limit (involvement of 25% of the entire white matter) to indicate when WML are to be considered severe.[69] Neuroimaging is also reputed today to allow a classification of the VaD into subtypes. The presence of extensive WML has been proposed as one of the two radiologic requirements for defining subcortical VaD in clinical trials.[70] To allow a diagnosis of subcortical VaD, WML must extend well beyond the periventricular region to affect the deeper white-matter structures of the hemispheric white matter. To support a diagnosis of subcortical VaD, on either CT or MRI, WML must be accompanied by lacunar infarcts.[70,71] Because the presence of severe WML in demented patients is considered to be a marker of VaD, neuroimaging has become an important requirement for recent and ongoing clinical trials of new drugs in VaD. Since the interrater agreement on the visual evaluation of WML is not always satisfactory,[72] many of these trials have adopted a centralized evaluation of scans.

Limitations and future directions

Below, some of the possible limitations of the studies that have evaluated the role of WML in cognitive impairment will be outlined. Possible targets for future research will also be sketched.

Location and extension of white-matter lesions

While data showing an effect of WML on cognitive functions are accumulating, a lack of knowledge remains about whether the location of WML is important in determining intellectual deficits. Since the majority of studies have found that WML cause cognitive deficits in frontal lobe tasks, it would be intuitive to hypothesize that lesions located anteriorly are most relevant. In one study, only frontal WML were found to be associated with a test of word fluency in 46 patients affected by early AD ($n = 12$), mild cognitive impairment ($n = 24$), and subjective memory disorders ($n = 10$).[73] Yet, this aspect remains to be fully demonstrated.

The results of other studies suggest that the volume of WML also has an impact on the possible neuropsychological correlates of these changes. In one study performed on healthy elderly patients, a threshold area for cognitive dysfunction was defined.[28] This observation was in line with the previous finding that the mean WML area in demented stroke patients was 10 times greater than in nondemented patients.[47] These studies underline the importance of a quantitative approach to the study of WML. In this sense, computerized WML evaluation, although more costly and time-consuming than visual evaluation, may prove unavoidable.[74,75]

Role of concurrent brain lesions

Many studies that have evaluated the possible role of WML in determining cognitive impairment lacked an assessment of the possible confounding effect of other brain changes that frequently coexist with WML. Among these changes, the most important appear to be cortical and/or hippocampal atrophy, lacunar infarcts, ventricular enlargement, and corpus callosum atrophy. Only more recently has this issue been taken into account in targeted studies. Mungas and coworkers evaluated a group of 157 patients with different neuropsychological profiles and heterogeneous clinical diagnoses, to detect

MRI correlates of cognitive scores.[76] They found that WML were associated with executive cognitive functions independently of other variables. However, the strongest predictors of cognitive performances were the volumes of cortical gray matter and the hippocampus. These results held true for patients both with and without subcortical lacunes. Yamauchi et al tested 62 patients with MMSE and a test of verbal fluency.[77] They found that, in the multivariate analysis, corpus callosum size was correlated with MMSE scores, while the extent of WML predicted the score of the verbal fluency task. These results are in line with those of other studies that found a correlation between WML and frontal lobe tasks. However, this study does not tell us whether a correlation also exists with other cognitive functions, because only two cognitive tests were applied. One interesting approach is that taken by Cook et al,[78] who evaluated in an integrated way the extension of structural brain changes, such as cortical atrophy, ventricular enlargement, and periventricular and deep white-matter hyperintensities (globally defined as subclinical structural brain disease), in relation to cognitive performances in 43 community-dwelling healthy subjects. They found that, although within the range of normal testing scores, small volumes of these subclinical structural brain changes also correlated with lower performances, particularly in frontal function tests.[78] Although these studies were performed in nondemented patients, it is likely that similar conclusions can be drawn for demented patients.

Assessment of noncognitive dysfunction linked to white-matter lesions

Limiting the assessment of the dysfunction associated with the presence and the severity of WML to the examination of cognitive deficits is probably too restricted. WML have, in fact, been found to be associated with motor dysfunction,[79] urinary incontinence,[80] and depressive symptoms;[81] therefore, the impact that the presence of these radiologic changes has on disability in the elderly may go well beyond that sustained by cognitive dysfunction. To assess specifically the risk of the transition to disability in subjects with various degrees of WML is the aim of one multicenter European collaborative study supported by the European Commission and coordinated by the Department of Neurological and Psychiatric Sciences of the University of Florence. The LADIS (Leukoaraiosis And Disability) study will prospectively assess over 700 nondisabled patients by means of cognitive, mood, and motor performance tests, and will correlate these with MRI findings and disability profiles.

Role of new magnetic resonance techniques

Some of the currently unsolved problems in the comprehension of the relation between WML and cognitive impairment may find possible solutions by the application of the MR techniques that have recently become available.

O'Sullivan and coworkers have applied diffusion tensor MRI to study possible ultrastructural brain abnormalities in 20 elderly subjects and 10 younger controls. All the subjects had normal conventional MRI, but diffusional anistropy, a marker of white-matter integrity, was reduced in the white matter of elderly subjects as age increased, indicating the loss of the normally packed structure of white-matter bundles.[82] Moreover, these authors were able to detect a correlation between the changes in diffusivity in the anterior white matter and executive dysfunction, as measured by the Trail Making Test.[82] The results of this study have been interpreted as supportive of the hypothesis of 'disconnection' as a possible mechanism of cognitive decline in the elderly without evident cortical damage. This hypothesis has found corroboration in another study that showed lower functional connectivity (as measured by EEG coherence) in patients with higher WML volumes.[78] By allowing the recognition of changes undetectable by conventional studies, the new MRI techniques might also shed some light on the role of WML in specific diseases. In one study performed in a small group of AD patients, diffusion changes of the white matter were found to correlate with MMSE score.[83]

Conclusions

The review of the studies that have evaluated the relation between WML and cognitive impairment showed strong consistency in the association of these radiologically detected changes with poorer performance in executive tasks and tests that depend on the integrity of the subcortical-frontal circuits. However, few doubts remain that the presence of WML poorly correlates with global cognitive performances and with scores of neuropsychological tests focused on memory functions. Although usually more prevalent and severe in VaD than in other disease conditions, WML are not, with few exceptions, to be considered the sole radiologic correlate of VaD. Still, when severe and associated with other specific clinical features, WML are one of the two hallmarks of subcortical VaD. It is also proposed that a proportion of nondisabled patients showing WML at baseline will develop a disabling condition that is partly due to cognitive impairment. Ongoing studies will clarify the details of this transition.

References

1. Inzitari D, Romanelli M, Pantoni L. Leukoaraiosis and cognitive impairment. In: O'Brien J, Ames D, Burns A, eds. Dementia, 2nd edn. London: Edward Arnold, 2000: 635–653.

2. Gunning-Dixon FM, Raz N. The cognitive correlates of white matter abnormalities in normal aging: a quantitative review. Neuropsychology 2000; 14: 224–232.

3. Inzitari D. Age-related white matter changes and cognitive impairment. Ann Neurol 2000; 47:141–143.

4. Ferro JM, Madureira S. Age-related white matter changes and cognitive impairment. J Neurol Sci 2002; 203–204:221–225.

5. Inzitari D, Diaz F, Fox A et al. Vascular risk factors and leuko-araiosis. Arch Neurol 1987; 44: 42–47.

6. Steingart A, Hachinski VC, Lau C et al. Cognitive and neurologic findings in demented patients with diffuse white matter lucencies on computed tomographic scan (leukoaraiosis). Arch Neurol 1987; 44:36–39.

7. Johnson KA, Davis KR, Buonanno FS et al. Comparison of magnetic resonance and roentgen ray computed tomography in dementia. Arch Neurol 1987; 44:1075–1080.

8. Diaz JF, Merskey H, Hachinski VC et al. Improved recognition of leukoaraiosis and cognitive impairment in Alzheimer's disease. Arch Neurol 1991; 48:1022–1025.

9. Lopez OL, Becker JT, Rezek D et al. Neuropsychiatric correlates of cerebral white-matter radiolucencies in probable Alzheimer's disease. Arch Neurol 1992; 49:828–834.

10. Skoog I, Berg S, Johansson B et al. The influence of white matter lesions on neuropsychological functioning in demented and non-demented 85-year-olds. Acta Neurol Scand 1996; 93:142–148.

11. Amar K, Bucks RS, Lewis T et al. The effect of white matter low attenuation on cognitive performance in dementia of the Alzheimer type. Age Ageing 1996; 25:443–448.

12. Fazekas F, Chawluk JB, Alavi et al. MR signal abnormalities at 1.5 T in Alzheimer's dementia and normal aging. Am J Neuroradiol AJNR 1987; 8:421–426.

13. Kertesz A, Polk M, Carr T. Cognition and white matter changes on magnetic resonance imaging in dementia. Arch Neurol 1990; 47:387–391.

14. Kozachuk WE, DeCarli C, Schapiro MB et al. White matter hyperintensities in dementia of Alzheimer's type and in healthy subjects without cerebrovascular risk factors. A magnetic resonance imaging study. Arch Neurol 1990; 47:1306–1310.

15. Bondareff W, Raval J, Woo B et al. Magnetic resonance imaging and the severity of dementia in older adults. Arch Gen Psychiatry 1990; 47:47–51.

16. Libon DJ, Scanlon M, Swenson R, Coslet HB. Binswanger's disease: some neuropsychological considerations. J Geriatr Psychiatry Neurol 1990; 3:31–40.

17. Leys D, Soetaert G, Petit H et al. Periventricular and white matter magnetic resonance imaging hyperintensities do not differ between Alzheimer's disease and normal aging. Arch Neurol 1990; 47:524–527.

18. Bowen BC, Barker WW, Loewenstein DA et al. MR signal abnormalities in memory disorders and dementia. Am J Neuroradiol AJNR 1990; 11:283–290.

19. Harrell LE, Duvall E, Folks DG et al. The relationship of high-intensity signals on magnetic resonance images to cognitive and psychiatric state in Alzheimer's disease. Arch Neurol 1991; 48:1136–1140.

20. Mirsen TR, Lee DH, Wong CJ et al. Clinical correlates of white-matter changes on magnetic resonance imaging scans of the brain. Arch Neurol 1991; 48:1015–1021.

21. McDonald WM, Krishnan KRR, Doraiswamy PM et al. Magnetic resonance findings in patients with early-onset Alzheimer's disease. Biol Psychiatry 1991; 29:799–810.

22. Almkvist O, Wahlund L-O, Andersson-Lundman G et al. White-matter hyperintensity and neuropsychological functions in dementia and healthy aging. Arch Neurol 1992; 49:626–632.

23. Bennett DA, Gilley DW, Wilson RS et al. Clinical correlates of high signal lesions on magnetic resonance imaging in Alzheimer's disease. J Neurol 1992; 239:186–190.

24. Marder K, Richards M, Bello J et al. Clinical correlates of Alzheimer's disease with and without silent radiographic abnormalities. Arch Neurol 1995; 52:146–151.

25. O'Brien J, Desmond P, Ames D et al. A magnetic resonance imaging study of white matter lesions in depression and Alzheimer's disease. Br J Psychiatry 1996; 168:477–485.

26. Stout JC, Jernigan TL, Archibald SL, Salmon DP. Association of dementia severity with cortical gray matter and abnormal white matter volumes in dementia of the Alzheimer type. Arch Neurol 1996; 53:742–749.

27. Starkstein SE, Sabe L, Vazquez S et al. Neuropsychological, psychiatric, and cerebral perfusion correlates of leukoaraiosis in Alzheimer's disease. J Neurol Neurosurg Psychiatry 1997; 63:66–73.

28. Boone KB, Miller BL, Lesser IM et al. Neuropsychological correlates of white-matter lesions in healthy elderly subjects. A threshold effect. Arch Neurol 1992; 49:549–554.

29. Ylikoski R, Ylikoski A, Erkinjuntti T et al. White matter changes in healthy elderly persons correlate with attention and speed of mental processing. Arch Neurol 1993; 50:818–824.

30. Schmidt R, Fazekas F, Offenbacher H et al. Neuropsychological correlates of MRI white matter hyperintensities: a study of 150 normal volunteers. Neurology 1993; 43:2490–2494.

31. Matsubayashi K, Shimada K, Kawamoto A, Ozawa T. Incidental brain lesions on magnetic resonance imaging and neurobehavioral functions in the apparently healthy elderly. Stroke 1992; 23:175–180.

32. Baum KA, Schulte C, Girke W et al. Incidental white-matter foci on MRI in 'healthy' subjects: evidence of subtle cognitive dysfunction. Neuroradiology 1996; 38:755–760.

33. Fukui T, Sugita K, Sato Y et al. Cognitive functions in subjects with incidental cerebral hyperintensities. Eur Neurol 1994; 34:272–276.

34. Breteler MMB, van Amerongen NM, van Swieten JC et al. Cognitive correlates of ventricular enlargement and cerebral white matter lesions on magnetic resonance imaging: the Rotterdam Study. Stroke 1994; 25:1109–1015.

35. Longstreth WT, Manolio TA, Arnold A et al. Clinical correlates of white matter findings on cranial magnetic resonance imaging of 3301 elderly people. The Cardiovascular Health Study. Stroke 1996; 267:1274–1282.

36. Fazekas F, Schmidt R, Roob G, Kapeller P. White matter changes in dementia. In: Leys D, Pasquier F, Scheltens Ph, eds. Stroke and Alzheimer's Disease. The Hague: Holland Academic Graphics, 1998: 183–195.

37. Smith CD, Snowdon DA, Wang H, Markesbery WR. White matter volumes and periventricular white matter hyperintensities in aging and dementia. Neurology 2000; 54:838–842.

38. Brun A, Englund E. A white matter disorder in dementia of the Alzheimer type: a pathoanatomical study. Ann Neurol 1986; 19:253–262.

39. Pantoni L, Garcia JH. Pathogenesis of leukoaraiosis: a review. Stroke 1997; 28:652–659.

40. Kalaria RN, Ballard C. Overlap between pathology of Alzheimer disease and vascular dementia. Alzheimer Dis Assoc Disord 1999; 13 (Suppl 3):S115–123.

41. de la Torre JC. Alzheimer disease as a vascular disorder: nosological evidence. Stroke 2002; 33:1152–1162.

42. Pantoni L. Pathophysiology of age-related cerebral white matter changes. Cerebrovasc Dis 2002; 13 (Suppl 2):7–10.

43. Scheltens P, Barkhof F, Valk J et al. White matter lesions on magnetic resonance imaging in clinically diagnosed Alzheimer's disease. Evidence for heterogeneity. Brain 1992; 115:735–738.

44. Fazekas F, Kapeller P, Schmidt R et al. The relation of cerebral magnetic resonance signal hyperintensities to Alzheimer's disease. J Neurol Sci 1996; 142:121–125.

45. Hirono N, Kitagaki H, Kazui H et al. Impact of white matter changes on clinical manifestation of Alzheimer's disease: a quantitative study. Stroke 2000; 31:2182–2188.

46. Tatemichi TK, Foulkes MA, Mohr JP et al. Dementia in stroke survivors in the Stroke Data Bank Cohort. Prevalence, incidence, risk factors, and computed tomographic findings. Stroke 1990; 21:858–866.

47. Liu CK, Miller BL, Cummings JL et al. A quantitative MRI study of vascular dementia. Neurology 1992; 42:138–143.

48. Censori B, Manara O, Agostinis C et al. Dementia after first stroke. Stroke 1996; 27:1205–1210.

49. Kase CS, Wolf PA, Kelly-Hayes M et al. Intellectual decline after stroke: the Framingham Study. Stroke 1998; 29:805–812.

50. Miyao S, Takano A, Teramoto J, Takahashi A. Leukoaraiosis in relation to prognosis for patients with lacunar infarction. Stroke 1992; 23:1434–1438.

51. Loeb C, Gandolfo C, Croce R, Conti M. Dementia associated with lacunar infarction. Stroke 1992; 23:1225–1229.

52. Henon H, Pasquier F, Durieu I et al. Preexisting dementia in stroke patients. Baseline frequency, associated factors, and outcome. Stroke 1997; 28:2429–2436.

53. Pohjasvaara T, Mäntylä R, Salonen O et al. How complex interactions of ischemic brain infarcts, white matter lesions, and atrophy relate to poststroke dementia. Arch Neurol 2000; 57:1295–1300.

54. Pohjasvaara T, Mäntylä R, Salonen O et al. MRI correlates of dementia

after first clinical ischemic stroke. J Neurol Sci 2000; 181:111–117.

55. Pantoni L, Leys D, Fazekas F et al. Role of white matter lesions in cognitive impairment of vascular origin. Alzheimer Dis Assoc Disord 1999; 13 (Suppl 3):S49–54.

56. Cummings JL. Frontal-subcortical circuits and human behavior. Arch Neurol 1993; 50:873–880.

57. Sultzer DL, Mahler ME, Cummings JL et al. Cortical abnormalities associated with subcortical lesions in vascular dementia. Clinical and position emission tomographic findings. Arch Neurol 1995; 52:773–780.

58. Wolf H, Ecke GM, Bettin S et al. Do white matter changes contribute to the subsequent development of dementia in patients with mild cognitive impairment? A longitudinal study. Int J Geriatr Psychiatry 2000; 15:803–812.

59. Vermeer SE, Prins ND, den Heijer T et al. Silent brain infarcts and the risk of dementia and cognitive decline. N Engl J Med 2003; 348:1215–1222.

60. Rockwood K, Wentzel C, Hachinski V et al. Prevalence and outcomes of vascular cognitive impairment. Vascular Cognitive Impairment Investigators of the Canadian Study of Health and Aging. Neurology 2000; 54:447–451.

61. Ebly EM, Hogan DB, Parhad IM. Cognitive impairment in the non-demented elderly. Results from the Canadian Study of Health and Aging. Arch Neurol 1995; 52:612–619.

62. Rockwood K. Vascular cognitive impairment and vascular dementia. J Neurol Sci 2002; 203–204:23–27.

63. Wentzel C, Rockwood K, MacKnight C et al. Progression of impairment in patients with vascular cognitive impairment without dementia. Neurology 2001; 57:714–716.

64. Ingles J, Wentzel C, Fisk JD, Rockwood K. Neuropsychological predictors of incident dementia in patients with vascular cognitive impairment, without dementia. Stroke 2002; 33:1999–2002.

65. Koga H, Yuzuriha T, Yao H et al. Quantitative MRI findings and cognitive impairment among community dwelling elderly subjects. J Neurol Neurosurg Psychiatry 2002; 72:737–741.

66. DeCarli C, Miller BL, Swan GE et al. Cerebrovascular and brain morphologic correlates of mild cognitive impairment in the National Heart, Lung, and Blood Institute Twin Study. Arch Neurol 2001; 58:643–647.

67. Erkinjuntti T, Ketonen L, Sulkava R et al. Do white matter changes on MRI and CT differentiate vascular dementia from Alzheimer's disease? J Neurol Neurosurg Psychiatry 1987; 50:37–42.

68. Pantoni L, Garcia JH. The significance of cerebral white matter abnormalities 100 years after Binswanger's report: a review. Stroke 1995; 26:1293–1301.

69. Román GC, Tatemichi TK, Erkinjuntti T et al. Vascular dementia: diagnostic criteria for research studies. Report of the NINDS–AIREN International Workshop. Neurology 1993; 43:250–260.

70. Erkinjuntti T, Inzitari D, Pantoni L et al. Research criteria for subcortical vascular dementia in clinical trials. J

Neural Trans Suppl 2000; 59:23–30.

71. Román GC, Erkinjuntti T, Wallin A et al. Subcortical ischaemic vascular dementia. Lancet Neurol 2002; 1:426–436.

72. Scheltens P, Erkinjuntti T, Leys D et al. White matter changes on CT and MRI: an overview of visual rating scales. European Task Force on Age-Related White Matter Changes. Eur Neurol 1998; 39:80–89.

73. Fernaeus SE, Almkvist O, Bronge L et al. White matter lesions impair initiation of FAS flow. Dement Geriatr Cogn Disord 2001; 12:52–56.

74. Pantoni L, Simoni M, Pracucci G et al. Visual rating scales for age-related white matter changes (leukoaraiosis): can the heterogeneity be reduced? Stroke 2002; 33:2827–2833.

75. Fazekas F, Barkhof F, Wahlund LO et al. CT and MRI rating of white matter lesions. Cerebrovasc Dis 2002; 13 (Suppl 2):31–36.

76. Mungas D, Jagust WJ, Reed BR et al. MRI predictors of cognition in subcortical ischemic vascular disease and Alzheimer's disease. Neurology 2001; 57:2229–2235.

77. Yamauchi H, Fukuyama H, Shio H. Corpus callosum atrophy in patients with leukoaraiosis may indicate global cognitive impairment. Stroke 2000; 31:1515–1520.

78. Cook IA, Leuchter AF, Morgan ML et al. Cognitive and physiologic correlates of subclinical structural brain disease in elderly healthy control subjects. Arch Neurol 2002; 59: 1612–1620.

79. Briley DP, Wasay M, Sergent S, Thomas S. Cerebral white matter changes (leukoaraiosis), stroke, and gait disturbance. J Am Geriatr Soc 1997; 45:1434–1438.

80. Sakakibara R, Hattori T, Uchiyama T, Yamanishi T. Urinary function in elderly people with and without leukoaraiosis: relation to cognitive and gait function. J Neurol Neurosurg Psychiatry 1999; 67:658–660.

81. de Groot JC, de Leeuw FE, Oudkerk M et al. Cerebral white matter lesions and depressive symptoms in elderly adults. Arch Gen Psychiatry 2000; 57:1071–1076.

82. O'Sullivan M, Summers PE, Jones DK et al. Normal-appearing white matter in ischemic leukoaraiosis: a diffusion tensor MRI study. Neurology 2001; 57:2307–2310.

83. Bozzali M, Falini A, Franceschi M et al. White matter damage in Alzheimer's disease assessed in vivo using diffusion tensor magnetic resonance imaging. J Neurol Neurosurg Psychiatry 2002; 72:742–746.

4
Subclassification of mild cognitive impairment in research and in clinical practice

Serge Gauthier and Jacques Touchon

Introduction

The concept of mild cognitive impairment (MCI) has been proposed by Petersen et al[1,2] as a nosologic entity referring to elderly persons with mild cognitive deficit without dementia. MCI is a seductive concept for clinicians and researchers because, unlike older concepts such as Age-Associated Memory Impairment (AAMI)[3] or Age-Associated Cognitive Decline (AACD),[4] it is assumed to be pathology-based and hence amenable to treatment or preventive actions. MCI is being widely used in epidemiologic and clinical studies as an intermediate stage between cognitive normality and dementia. A high number of persons have been found to suffer from MCI in the population at large, and many are now being referred to memory clinics. There is an expectation of even larger numbers of individuals with memory complaints coming forward for assessment as the results of the ongoing randomized clinical trials become available. MCI appears to be a heterogeneous clinical entity.[5] Multiple sources of heterogeneity have been described: heterogeneity in etiologic factors (various types of degenerative lesions, vascular lesions, psychiatric features, and association with nonneurologic pathologic conditions), heterogeneity in clinical symptoms,[6] and heterogeneity in clinical course.[7] The heterogeneity of MCI has been recognized,[8] and the first consensus report has recommended that the term 'MCI' be qualified by an appropriate modifier. We thus propose a subclassification of MCI for use in research and in clinical practice.

Mild cognitive impairment in population-based epidemiologic studies

Estimates of the prevalence of MCI in population-based epidemiologic studies vary greatly depending on the definition in use, ranging from 3% to 16.8%.[9] The former figure is obtained from specialized referral clinics using amnestic MCI criteria (see below), whereas the latter figure has been documented in the Canadian Study of Health and Aging, where the term 'cognitive impairment no dementia' (CIND) was defined as various categories of impairment identified in a clinical examination and neuro-psychological tests.[10] The most common cause of CIND was 'circumscribed memory impairment', a close equivalent of amnestic MCI, with a prevalence of 5.3%.[11] The follow-up of individuals with vascular CIND demonstrated that after 5 years 52% had died and 46% had developed dementia,[12] whereas MCI defined by different criteria led to a wide range of conversion to dementia (20.0–50.9%), AD (11.6–28.8%), and death (30.1–42.4%).[13]

A large-scale epidemiologic study based on a general practice research network in France (the Eugeria Study) revealed a prevalence of 3.2% for MCI.[7] The diagnostic criteria used for MCI were those initially proposed by Petersen et al.[1] including: 1) the presence of a subjective memory complaint, 2) preserved general intellectual functioning, 3) demonstration of a memory impairment by cognitive testing, 4) intact ability to perform activities of daily living (ADL), 5) absence of dementia. According to Petersen et al,[2] the subjects were impaired on a memory task only, and not on tests relating to other cognitive functions. Out of 833 subjects, 27 were classified as having MCI. MCI was a poor predictor of dementia within a 3-year period, with an 11.1% conversion rate. Subjects with MCI constituted an unstable group, with many subjects changing category each year during the 3-year follow-up. Many subjects reverted to normal cognition, and others remained stable.[7] In another cohort in France, out of 1265 subjects, 58 prevalent cases of MCI were observed at baseline, demonstrating a prevalence of 2.8%. During a 5-year follow-up, 40 incident cases of MCI occurred, and an annual conversion rate of 8.3% was observed. The MCI group was very unstable across time in this study. Within 2–3 years, only 6% of the subjects continued to have MCI, whereas more than 40% reverted to normal.[14]

The Kungsholmen Project is another population study looking at MCI, in which a subclassification was made within CIND of mild, moderate, or severe based on Mini-Mental State Examination scores (MMSE) (mild: 1 SD below age- and education-specific mean scores; moderate: 1.5 SD; severe: 2 SD). Depression and cerebrovascular disease were more common in the CIND population than in unimpaired subjects; similar proportions of CIND subjects progressed to dementia, death, and cognitive improvement over 3 years.[15] In the Eugeria Study, the prevalence of depressive symptoms and depressive illness was higher in elderly people with subclinical cognitive impairment than in the general population (76% reporting at least one depressive symptom).[16]

In a cross-sectional study derived from the Cardiovascular Health Study,[17] the NPI (NeuroPsychiatric Inventory) was used to define the presence and severity of neuropsychiatric symptoms in MCI: 43% of MCI subjects exhibited neuropsychiatric symptoms, depression (20%), apathy (15%), and irritability (15%), being most common.

Table 4.1. Subclassification of MCI in specialized clinics.

Amnestic or single memory MCI
Multiple domain MCI
Single non-memory-domain MCI

MCI: mild cognitive impairment.

Mild cognitive impairment in specialty clinic-based observational studies

Specialized clinics in Rochester and St Louis have established that amnestic MCI is frequently a prodrome to AD[2] or its first manifestation.[18] The heterogeneity within MCI has been noted and a classification has been proposed (Table 4.1).[19]

The outcome of the different kinds of MCI is variable. According to Petersen et al,[6] subjects with amnestic MCI usually progress to AD, and subjects with multiple domain slightly impaired MCI could progress to AD or to vascular dementia, or they might represent normal aging. The outcome of single non-memory-domain MCI could be any of the following: frontotemporal dementia, Lewy body dementia, vascular dementia, primary progressive aphasia, Parkinson's disease, and AD.

To complicate matters, there appears to be clinical and pathologic heterogeneity even within amnestic MCI.[5]

Mild cognitive impairment in randomized clinical trials

The operational definition of amnestic MCI has made possible large-scale, placebo-controlled, randomized clinical trials (RCT) to test the hypothesis

Table 4.2. Subclassification of MCI in randomized clinical trials using cholinesterase inhibitors.

	Donepezil	Rivastigmine	Galantamine
Primary outcome	Conversion to AD	Conversion to AD	Symptomatic
Age (years)	55–90	55–85	50 and older
MMSE	> 23	–	–
Global CDR	0.5	0.5	0.5
NYU delayed paragraph recall	–	< 9	< 11
Logical memory II from Wechsler Memory Scale	< cutpoint adjusted for education	–	–
Hamilton	< 13	< 13	–

AD: Alzheimer's disease; MCI: mild cognitive impairment

Table 4.3. Operational clinical criteria for amnestic MCI in rofecoxib study.[14]

Subjects report memory problems, or informant reports that subject has memory problems

Informant reports that subject's memory has declined in the past year

MMSE > 23

Rey Auditory Verbal Learning Test score < 38

CDR global score 0.5 with memory domain score ≥0.5

Blessed ADL total score ≤3.5, with no part 1 item score > 0.5

that the treatment of MCI with a cholinesterase inhibitor (CI), such as donepezil, rivastigmine, or galantamine, can delay the diagnosis of AD and/or improve cognitive impairments. Slightly different MCI populations are defined for each study (Table 4.2).

Information is also available on the definition of MCI as used in therapy with the selective cyclooxygenase-2 inhibitor, rofecoxib, in attempting to delay conversion to AD (Table 4.3).[20]

Other issues about RCT for MCI have been reviewed by Geda and Petersen, including the potential value of neuroimaging as a surrogate outcome.[21] One of the galantamine MCI studies includes whole-brain volumetric measurements at baseline, and 1- and 2-year visits as a secondary outcome.

Mild cognitive impairment at higher risk of progression to dementia

There are patterns of risk emerging from general-population epidemiologic studies, clinical observations, and RCT for higher risks of progression. It is likely that models combining multiple risk factors, such as the ones listed in Table 4.4, will be needed to predict the risk of individuals with MCI progressing to dementia.[22–30]

There is no consensus concerning brain imaging in MCI. However, both morphologic and functional imaging may facilitate diagnosis, particularly with regard to the differentiation of subtypes of MCI and the identification of prodromal AD. Hypoactivity shown by PET or SPECT, within structures affected early in AD, such as the temporal lobe and the posterior cingulate gyrus, could have a diagnostic utility.[31,32]

Increase in cerebrospinal fluid tau and decrease in Aβ42 have been proposed as predictors of the development of AD in patients with MCI.[33] The phosphorylated tau:total tau ratio could be more accurate for the diagnosis.

Table 4.4. Subclassification of amnestic MCI at higher risk of progression to dementia.

Poor performance on delayed recall and executive function tests[23,24]

Carer's report of 1) impaired daily function,[25] particularly for ability to use the telephone, mode of transportation, responsibility for own medication, ability to handle finances;[26] 2) changes in abilities over the past year using a proxy screening questionnaire (activity level, semantic and visual memory, memory for places, events, and procedures, visuospatial performances and new skill learning)[27]

Hippocampal atrophy (2.5 SD below norms for age and sex)[28]

APOE4 genotype[29]

Midlife vascular risk factors[30]

These markers will be especially important when drugs with effect on the progression of AD become available.

Mild cognitive impairment in clinical practice

In clinical practice, the association of neuropsychological evaluation and collateral source reports are necessary to detect the subtle cognitive and functional decline that characterizes MCI. The following diagnostic criteria for MCI could be proposed:

1) subject's report of cognitive problems, or informant report that subject has cognitive problems
2) informant report of a history of decline in cognitive and functional performances in the past year, in relation to that patient's previous abilities
3) preserved general intellectual functioning
4) demonstration of mild cognitive impairment by cognitive testing: memory impairment and/or impairment in other cognitive domains
5) mild difficulties in complex daily living activities
6) absence of dementia.

The heterogeneity of MCI implies the definition of different subtypes of MCI. A simple classification of MCI is proposed for use in clinical practice, based on the main subtypes of patients over age 50 commonly encountered in neurology referral practice (Table 4.5). The importance of neuropsychiatric symptoms in MCI is starting to emerge from systematic studies using the NPI, depression, apathy, and irritability being most common[17] (see also Chapter 5). In our experience, this is the most common type of MCI, which we label 'dysthymic'. The second most common is 'vascular', as found in cognitive impairment associated with vascular risk factors such as systolic hypertension, diabetes mellitus, hypercholesterolemia, and white-matter changes

Table 4.5. Subclassification of MCI for clinical practice.

Dysthymic
Vascular
Amnestic
Miscellaneous

and/or lacunae on brain imaging. Less common is 'amnestic', defined as memory-only complaints, lack of vascular clinical or radiologic features, and absence of depressive features. A 'miscellaneous' category could include other causes such as alcohol abuse, sedative and anticholinergic drug abuse, metabolic and nutritional deficiencies, and sleep apnea syndrome.

Since the depressive or 'dysthymic MCI' profile may represent a prodrome to dementia[34] or even subclinical AD,[35] yearly follow-up visits are suggested, in addition to treating depressive symptoms with a SSRI or other relevant drug and/or supportive psychotherapy. Although less likely to deteriorate over time, 'vascular MCI' requires treatment and follow-up of the associated conditions. Finally, 'amnestic MCI' requires follow-up until dementia is diagnosable, at which time a CI can be prescribed. The preliminary results of a 24-week, randomized study comparing donepezil with placebo in amnestic MCI revealed minimal benefit and high dropout rates,[36] suggesting that this class of drug is better used when AD is diagnosable. This minimal benefit of CI in MCI could be explained by an upregulation of choline acetyltransferase activity.[37] DeKosky et al[37] have shown that inferior parietal, superior temporal, and cingulate cortices choline acetyltransferase activity was unchanged in subjects with MCI and mild AD when compared with normal controls. Furthermore hippocampal choline acetyltransferase activity was higher in MCI subjects than in normal controls. According to these results, the rationale of cholinergic treatment in MCI is not well established. In amnestic MCI, other brain changes besides cholinergic hypofunction, could be implied.

In MCI therapeutic strategies, the role of anti-inflammatory drugs, hormonal replacement therapy, antioxidant agents, and glutamatergic drugs remains to be demonstrated.

Conclusions

The study of the different subtypes of MCI offers an opportunity to understand the natural history of cognitive changes with age, and the potential for prevention of dementia, particularly the AD type. Directions for future research should include the definition of prodromal states for non-AD dementias, potentially leading to secondary prevention. Also in need of clarification is the distinction between mild but potentially significant high-order ADL impairment in MCI, such as financial capacity,[38] versus early diagnosable dementia.

Of pressing urgency is the confirmation that there are predictors for progression from amnestic MCI to dementia that can be used by clinicians to detect those among the forgetful patients that need early pharmacologic treatment. Guidelines such as those developed by the American Academy of Neurology[1] will need to be updated periodically, as new evidence on the natural history of amnestic and other types of MCI, and hopefully stabilization approaches, become available.

To help resolve the uncertainty of the operational definitions of MCI in clinical practice, as well as help regulators deal with an entity not clearly recognized in the DSM and other evidence- and consensus-based diagnostic criteria, the notion of 'prodromal AD', as proposed by Dubois,[39] may prove very useful, since experienced clinicians understand this concept. Defining which cases of MCI are prodromal AD is a preliminary condition for the development of novel therapeutic strategies. An update of the NINCDS–ADRDA criteria[40] could incorporate this notion of prodromal or very early stage of AD.

References

1. Petersen RC, Smith GE, Waring SC et al. Aging, memory and mild cognitive impairment. Int Psychogeriatr 1997; 9:65–69.

2. Petersen RC, Smith GE, Waring SC et al. Mild clinical impairment: clinical characterization and outcome. Arch Neurol 1999; 56:303–308.

3. Crook T, Bartus RT, Ferris SH et al. Age associated memory impairment: proposed diagnostic criteria and measures of clinical change: report of the National Institute of Mental Health Work Group. Dev Neuropsychol 1986; 2:261–276.

4. Levy R, on behalf of the Aging-Associated Cognitive Decline Working Party. Aging-associated cognitive decline. Int Psychogeriatr 1994; 6:63–68.

5. Lautenschlager NT, Riemenschneider M, Drzezga A, Kurz AF. Primary degenerative mild cognitive impairment: study population, clinical, brain imaging and biochemical findings. Dement Geriatr Cogn Disord 2001; 12:379–386.

6. Petersen RC, Doody R, Kurz A et al. Current concepts in mild cognitive impairment. Arch Neurol 2001; 58:1985–1992.

7. Ritchie K, Artero S, Touchon J. Classification criteria for mild cognitive impairment. A population-based validation study. Neurology 2001; 56:37–42.

8. Petersen RC, Stevens JC, Ganguli M et al. Practice parameter: early detection of dementia: mild cognitive impairment (an evidence-based review). Report of the Quality Standards Subcommittee of the American Academy of Neurology. Neurology 2001; 56:1133–1142.

9. DeCarli C. Mild cognitive impairment: prevalence, prognosis, aetiology, and treatment. Lancet Neurol 2003; 2:15–21.

10. Graham JE, Rockwood K, Beattie BL et al. Standardization of the diagnosis of dementia in the Canadian Study of Health and Aging. Neuroepidemiology 1996; 15:246–256.

11. Graham JE, Rockwood K, Beattie BL et al. Prevalence and severity of cognitive impairment with and without dementia in an elderly population. Lancet 1997; 349: 1793–1796.

12. Wentzel C, Rockwood K, MacKnight C et al. Neurology 2001; 57:714–716.

13. Hogan DB, Ebly EM. Predicting who will develop dementia in a cohort of Canadian seniors. Can J Neurol Sci 2000; 27:18–24.

14. Larrieu S, Letenneur L, Orgogozo JM et al. Incidence and outcome of mild cognitive impairment in a population-based prospective cohort. Neurology 2002; 59:1594–1599.

15. Palmer K, Wang HX, Winblad B, Fratiglioni L. Differential evolution of cognitive impairment in nondemented older persons: results from the Kungsholmen Project. Am J Psychiatry 2002; 159:436–442.

16. Ritchie K, Guilham C, Ledesert B et al. Depressive illness, depressive symptomatology and regional cerebral blood flow in elderly with sub-clinical cognitive impairment. Age Ageing 1999; 28:385–391.

17. Lyketsos CG, Lopez O, Jones B et al. Prevalence of neuropsychiatric symptoms in dementia and mild cognitive impairment. JAMA 2002; 288:1475–1483.

18. Morris JC, Storandt M, Miller JP et al. Mild cognitive impairment represents early-stage Alzheimer's disease. Arch Neurol 2001; 58: 397–405.

19. Petersen RC. Conceptual overview. In: Petersen RC, ed. Mild Cognitive Impairment: Aging to Alzheimer's Disease. New York: Oxford University Press, 2003; 1–14.

20. Lines CR, McCarroll A, Lipton RB, Block GA, on behalf of the Prevention of Alzheimer's in Society's Elderly Study Group. Neurology 2003; 60:261–266.

21. Geda YE, Petersen RC. Clinical trials in mild cognitive impairment. In: Gauthier S, Cummings JL, eds. Alzheimer's Disease and Related Disorders Annual 2001. London: Martin Dunitz, 2001:69–83.

22. Marquis S, Moore MM, Howieson DB et al. Independent predictors of cognitive decline in healthy elderly persons. Arch Neurol 2002; 59:601–606.

23. Chen P, Ratcliff G, Belle SH et al. Cognitive tests that best discriminate between presymptomatic AD and those who remain nondemented. Neurology 2000; 55:1847–1853.

24. Ritchie K, Touchon J. Prodromal cognitive disorder in Alzheimer's disease. Int J Geriatr Psychiatry 1999; 14:556–563.

25. Tabert MH, Albert SM, Borukhova-Milov L et al. Functional deficits in patients with mild cognitive impairment. Prediction of AD. Neurology 2002; 58:758–764.

26. Barberger-Gateau P, Fabrigoule C, Helmer C et al. Functional impairment in instrumental activities of daily living: an early clinical sign of dementia? J Am Geriatr Soc 1999; 47:456–462.

27. Ritchie K, Fuhrer R. The validation of an informant screening test for irreversible cognitive decline in the elderly: performance characteristics

within a general population sample. Int J Geriatr Psychiatry 1996; 11:149–156.

28. Jack CR, Petersen RC, Xu YC et al. Prediction of AD with MRI-based hippocampal volume in mild cognitive impairment. Neurology 1999; 52:1397–1403.

29. Dik MG, Jonker C, Comijs HC et al. Memory complaints and APOE-epsilon 4 accelerate cognitive decline in cognitively normal elderly. Neurology 2001; 57:2217–2222.

30. Kivipelto M, Helkala EL, Hänninen T et al. Midlife vascular risk factors and late-life mild cognitive impairment. A population-based study. Neurology 2001; 56: 1683–1689.

31. Johnson KA, Jones K, Holman BL et al. Preclinical prediction of Alzheimer's disease using SPECT. Neurology 1998; 50:1563–1571.

32. De Leon MJ, Convit A, Wolf OT et al. Prediction of cognitive decline in normal elderly subjects with 2-[(18)F]fluoro-2-deoxy-D-glucose/positron-emission tomography (FDG/PET). Proc Natl Acad Sci USA 2001; 98:10966–10971.

33. Andreasen N, Vanmechelen E, Vanderstichele H et al. Cerebrospinal fluid levels of total-tau, phospho-tau and A beta 42 predict development of Alzheimer's disease in patients with mild cognitive impairment. Acta Neurol Scand Suppl 2003; 179:47–51.

34. Schweitzer I, Tuckwell V, O'Brien J, Ames D. Is late onset depression a prodrome to dementia? Int J Geriatr Psychiatry 2002; 17:997–1005.

35. Geerlings MI, Schmand B, Braam AW et al. Depressive symptoms and risk of Alzheimer's disease in more highly educated older people. J Am Geriatr Soc 2000; 48: 1092–1097.

36. Salloway SP, Kumar D, Ieni J et al. Benefits of donepezil treatment in patients with mild cognitive impairment. Neurology 2003; 60(Suppl 1):A411–412.

37. DeKosky ST, Ikonomovic MD, Styren SD et al. Upregulation of choline acetyltransferase activity in hippocampus and frontal cortex of elderly subjects with mild cognitive impairment. Ann Neurol 2002; 51:145–155.

38. Griffith HR, Belue K, Sicola A et al. Impaired financial abilities in mild cognitive impairment. A direct assessment approach. Neurology 2003; 60:449–457.

39. Dubois B. 'Prodromal Alzheimer's disease': a more useful concept than mild cognitive impairment? Curr Opin Neurol 2000; 13:367–369.

40. McKhann G, Drachman D, Folstein M et al. Clinical diagnosis of Alzheimer's disease: report of the NINCDS–ADRDA Work Group under the auspices of Department of Health and Human Services Task Force on Alzheimer's Disease. Neurology 1984; 34:939–944.

5
Neuropsychiatric symptoms of mild cognitive impairment

Tzung J Hwang and Jeffrey L Cummings

Neuropsychiatric symptoms are common in patients with dementia or Alzheimer's disease (AD).[1–3] They include a broad range of symptoms from apathy, agitation, mood symptoms (dysphoria and anxiety), psychosis (delusions and hallucinations), to sleep and appetite disturbances. Some symptoms are clustered into syndromes, and provisional operational criteria, such as AD-related psychosis or depression, are proposed to facilitate their study.[4,5] These symptoms have serious negative consequences for patients, including compromising quality of life and increasing impairment in activities of daily living. They are also major sources of psychological stress, depression, and burden for the caregivers.[6] Studies have shown that these symptoms are linked to elder abuse and are important determinants of the institutionalization of patients with AD.[7,8] Neuropsychiatric symptoms reflect the underlying neurobiological changes of the diseased brain, and many can be alleviated by psychotropic medications.[9,10] Certain stage-specific patterns of the neuropsychiatric symptoms can be observed during the course of AD,[11] and some symptoms may have specific value in the prediction of the disease course. For example, several studies have found that depression is a harbinger of AD;[12,13] others have shown that delusions or hallucinations predict clinical or functional decline.[14,15]

Mild cognitive impairment (MCI) describes cognitive impairment in the elderly not of sufficient severity to meet diagnostic criteria for dementia. It is often a transitional state between normal aging and dementia. Subjects with MCI have memory impairment or other cognitive deficits that may be noticeable to their family. Objective cognitive tests show worse performance than their age- and education-comparable contemporaries. However, their daily function is generally preserved.

Many terms have been applied in the literature to describe MCI in the elderly population. Although sharing a certain similarity, each term has its own concept and definition, and encompasses a specific group of subjects.

MCI may be a precursor to dementia.[16,17] The reported annual conversion rates to AD are 1–25% per year, depending on different definitions of MCI and different populations studied.[18] Certain types of MCI have higher conversion rates. For example, the amnestic MCI as defined by Petersen et al's criteria[16] has an annual conversion rate of 10–15%, compared with that of 1–2% in healthy controls.[16,19] Neuroimaging studies have shown that hippocampal atrophy in amnestic MCI is greater than that in controls, and this finding is predictive of subsequent conversion to AD.[20] Proton magnetic resonance spectroscopy and cerebrospinal fluid (CSF) studies also suggest that MCI is distinct from normal aging and bears features similar to those of AD.[21–23] These results indicate that the neurobiological changes in MCI, at least in certain kinds of MCI, are less severe than but similar to those of AD. Similarly, neuropsychiatric symptoms associated with AD may be anticipated in MCI.

Few studies have focused on the neuropsychiatric symptoms in subjects with MCI, but the study of these symptoms is important for three reasons. First, the present provisional diagnostic criteria of MCI depend mainly on cognitive functioning and do not include noncognitive neuropsychiatric symptoms, which may also be important features of this condition. Characterization of these symptoms may have diagnostic value or definitional implications in MCI. Second, since neuropsychiatric symptoms are likely to be associated with underlying pathophysiological changes in the brain, studying these symptoms can help to understand the nature of MCI. Third, some of these symptoms, like those in AD, may have predictive or prognostic values in the course of MCI, and thus merit investigation.

The purpose of this chapter is to review the available data on the neuropsychiatric symptoms of MCI, and discuss possible neurobiological bases of these symptoms.

Different definitions of mild cognitive impairment

Different studies on neuropsychiatric symptoms may be based on different definitions, encompassing subjects with different characteristics. Among them, amnestic MCI by Petersen's criteria[16] and 'cognitive impairment, no dementia' (CIND) are increasingly important. Amnestic MCI emphasizes isolated memory impairment (a subjective memory complaint and objective memory test performance deficit) with preserved general intellectual ability and daily function, and without dementia. In contrast, the diagnosis of CIND is based on the absence of dementia and the presence of various cognitive impairments identified in the clinical examination and neuropsychological tests. The subcategories of CIND include medical and psychiatric illness such as delirium, chronic alcohol and drug use, depression, mental retardation, and subclinical dementia. Thus, the concept of CIND implies a broader range of cognitive pathology than that of MCI. Other concepts designating cognitive impairment in elderly people without dementia include benign senescent forgetfulness, age-associated memory impairment, late-life forgetfulness, age-associated cognitive decline, age-related cognitive decline, mild cognitive disorder, and mild neurocognitive disorder. All these concepts are different from each other, and the validity of these concepts is still under investigation.[18] Since data on neuropsychiatric symptoms of MCI are available only on amnestic MCI and CIND, this review will focus on the research findings of neuropsychiatric features related to these two concepts.

Assessment of neuropsychiatric symptoms

Characterization of neuropsychiatric symptoms requires appropriate instrumentation. One of the tools most frequently used for the purpose in dementia research is the Neuropsychiatric Inventory (NPI).[24] Developed in 1994, this instrument assesses 12 types of neuropsychiatric disturbances common in dementia, including delusions, hallucinations, agitation, dysphoria, anxiety, apathy, irritability, euphoria, disinhibition, aberrant motor behavior, nighttime behavior disturbances, and appetite and eating abnormalities. Severity and frequency are assessed separately. The administration of the NPI is based on a structured interview with a caregiver who is familiar with the patient. A screening question for each domain is asked first, followed by a set of subquestions if the response to the screening question suggests the presence of behavioral changes in that domain. After administration of subquestions, the caregiver is asked to rate the severity on a 3-point scale (1 = mild to 3 = severe) and frequency on a 4-point scale (1 = occasionally, less than once per week to 4 = very frequently, one or more per day, or continuously) of each abnormality. Each rating is scripted with detailed anchor points. A score for the individual domain is calculated by multiplying the severity by the frequency. In addition to a score for the individual symptom domain, a total NPI score is calculated by summing the individual scores. The interrater reliability, test–retest reliability, content validity, and concurrent validity of the NPI are established.[24] The NPI has been used to assess patients with MCI, and the results discussed here will emphasize findings emerging with the use of this instrument.

Neuropsychiatric symptoms of mild cognitive impairment

There are three recent studies with available data on the neuropsychiatric symptoms of MCI. The first study has a clinical sample of amnestic MCI (n = 28) referred to the University of California, Los Angeles (UCLA) medical center. The second study has a clinical sample of CIND (n = 196) from a longitudinal cohort composed of referred subjects to eight dementia research centers across Canada. The third study is a population-based study with 320 subjects of CIND from four US communities. Thus, the characteristics of subjects in the three studies are different from one another. The percentage of subjects with neuropsychiatric symptoms in these studies is summarized in Table 5.1. Overall, the frequencies of neuropsychiatric symptoms in the clinical subjects of amnestic MCI were close to but somewhat less than those in the clinical subjects of CIND. In contrast, the frequencies of neuropsychiatric symptoms in the community subjects of CIND were substantially lower than those of the two clinical samples. These results also reflected on the total NPI scores, of which the clinical subjects of CIND had the highest (Table 5.1). Such results can be explained by the differences of characteristics among study subjects. Where clinical subjects are concerned, subjects with CIND have more severe neuropsychiatric symptoms than those with amnestic MCI, because CIND encompasses a broader range of cognitive deficits than amnestic MCI, which has only isolated memory impairment. Clinical subjects show higher prevalence rates of symptoms than community subjects since the former, in general, have greater severity of symptoms prompting clinical assessment. Clinical samples of subjects with amnestic MCI have a higher prevalence of almost all symptoms than community subjects with CIND, suggesting that the origin of subjects (referral versus community) outweighs the diagnostic subcategorization (amnestic MCI versus CIND) in their influence on the frequency and severity of neuropsychiatric symptoms.

When the prevalence of the 10 symptoms is examined, a similar pattern is observed in all three studies. Mood symptoms (dysphoria, irritability, and anxiety) and apathy are the most prevalent, followed by agitation, and then disinhibition/aberrant motor behavior. Delusions, hallucinations, and euphoria are the least prevalent. Table 5.2 shows the neuropsychiatric features of 50 normal controls, 28 amnestic MCI subjects, and 124 subjects with mild

Table 5.1. Percentage of neuropsychiatric symptoms and total NPI scores in three different samples (see text for reference).

	Clinical samples of amnestic MCI (n = 28)	Clinical samples of CIND (n = 196)	Community samples of CIND (n = 320)
	%	%	%
Hallucinations	0	4	1
Delusions	4	7	3
Agitation	18	23	11
Dysphoria	39	42	20
Anxiety	25	30	10
Euphoria	11	3	1
Apathy	39	37	15
Disinhibition	18	16	3
Irritability	29	39	15
Aberrant motor behavior	14	12	4
	Mean (SD)	Mean (SD)	Mean (SD)
NPI total scores	7.4 (8.4)	9.9 (15.1)	N/S

NPI: Neuropsychiatric Inventory; amnestic MCI: mild cognitive impairment by Petersen's criteria; CIND: cognitive impairment, no dementia; N/S: not specified.

AD (defined by a MMSE score of ≥ 21) assessed at UCLA. The pattern of neuropsychiatric symptoms in MCI was similar to that of mild AD (Table 5.2), but not similar to that reported in severe AD[2] when apathy, agitation, and aberrant motor behavior become predominate. In addition, in the UCLA study, although there were no significant differences in the proportion of patients manifesting neuropsychiatric symptoms between the amnestic MCI and mild AD subjects, the mild AD subjects were significantly more likely to have delusions than the amnestic MCI subjects. The findings from this study suggest that there is an evolution of the neuropsychiatric symptoms from a preclinical stage with mood symptoms to higher frequencies of psychotic symptoms after patients meet criteria for AD.

Mood abnormalities

The most significant neuropsychiatric symptoms of MCI are mood abnormalities. In a study on the natural history of 100 autopsy-confirmed AD patients, depression was shown to be present about 26 months before the diagnosis of AD, followed by psychotic symptoms, which occurred at about the same time as the diagnosis.[25] Another study of the psychopathology of very mild or questionable AD (Clinical Dementia Rating score $= 0.5$) made similar observations.[26] These studies indicate that depression may be a harbinger of AD. In addition to depression, other studies found that anxiety and irritability also were common in the early phase of AD.[2,11,27] Although mood

Table 5.2. Percentage of subjects with neuropsychiatric symptoms and total NPI scores in the control, MCI, and mild AD group in the UCLA study.

	Control (n = 50)		Amnestic MCI (n = 28)		Mild AD (n = 124)		MCI vs. control	MCI vs. mild AD
	n	%	n	%	n	%	p (Fisher's exact test)	
Hallucinations	0	0	0	0	7	6	NS	NS
Delusions	0	0	1	4	32	26	0.359	0.010
Agitation	0	0	5	18	42	34	0.005	0.116
Dysphoria	4	8	11	39	62	50	0.002	0.403
Anxiety	1	2	7	25	43	35	0.003	0.379
Euphoria	0	0	3	11	10	8	NS	NS
Apathy	1	2	11	39	63	51	0.000	0.301
Disinhibition	2	4	5	18	26	21	0.091	0.801
Irritability	2	4	8	29	47	38	0.003	0.392
Aberrant motor behavior	0	0	4	14	34	27	0.014	0.226
	Mean	SD	Mean	SD	Mean	SD	p (Dunnett T3)	
NPI total score	0.9	4.3	7.4	8.4	10.4	11.4	0.001	0.304

NS: $P > 0.05$ in the chi-square test among the three groups.
Mild AD is defined as a MMSE score of ≥ 21.

abnormalities may be a reactive psychological response to emerging cognitive deficits in subjects with MCI, this may not account entirely for their occurrence.

Neuropathologic studies have shown that the limbic system is involved in the early phases of AD.[28] Subjects with MCI may have neuropathologic changes of AD,[17] and the abnormalities are most severe in the limbic system.[29,30] Neuroimaging studies have indicated that limbic pathology is present in MCI.[20,22] Thus, mood abnormalities in MCI can be the manifestations of underlying neurobiological changes in the limbic system.

Apathy

Several studies have shown that apathy is among the most frequent neuropsychiatric symptoms in AD.[2,26,31] Neurobiological studies reveal that the cingulate gyrus plays an important role in apathy in AD and other neuropsychiatric disorders.[32–34] Early involvement of the limbic system (including the cingulate gyrus) in MCI may partially account for the appearance of apathy.

Depression and apathy are related. Although depression and apathy are not the same, they may be associated. Depressed patients usually, but do not necessarily, have decreased interest in daily activity and social interaction. In the UCLA study, the co-occurrence rate of dysphoria and apathy was 73% in subjects with amnestic MCI, and 64% in patients with mild AD. However, apathy can occur in the absence of depression. When AD becomes more severe, the correlation between apathy and depression may decline.[35] In an analysis of UCLA NPI data, of 270 patients with various degrees of AD (mild AD 135, moderate AD 97, and severe AD 38), the co-occurrence rate of dysphoria and apathy decreased from 64% in mild AD to 45% in severe AD, and the Spearman correlation between apathy and dysphoria scores changed from +0.320 to –0.135.

Psychosis

Psychotic symptoms are common in patients with AD.[36] The most common symptoms include persecutory delusions, misidentification syndromes, and hallucinations. A low prevalence of psychotic symptoms is found in subjects with MCI from both clinical or community samples (Table 5.1). Delusions tend to be more frequent than hallucinations. As the disease progresses, psychotic symptoms may significantly increase. In the UCLA study of clinical subjects with amnestic MCI and mild AD, delusions occurred in 4% of subjects with amnestic MCI, a percentage significantly less than the 26% in subjects with mild AD ($P = 0.01$) (Table 5.2). Hallucinations also increased from 0% in amnestic MCI to 7% in mild AD, but the difference was not significant ($P > 0.05$).

There is evidence that neurobiological changes may underly the appearance of psychotic symptoms in AD. Studies show that neurophysiological and neurochemical changes in frontal or temporal lobes are associated with psychotic symptoms in AD.[37–39] A large neuropathologic study showed that AD subjects with psychosis had a significantly greater burden of neocortical neurofibrillary tangles than those without.[40] Since MCI may have pathology limited to the limbic system, the low frequency of psychotic symptoms may reflect this restricted distribution of pathologic changes.

Discussion

Cognitive impairment without dementia has frequently been considered to be the result of the normal aging process. Several concepts have been proposed to define such a state, including benign senescent forgetfulness, age-associated memory impairment, age-associated cognitive decline, and age-related cognitive decline. These concepts consider mild cognitive deficits to be a variant of normal aging. Another line of thinking considers mild cognitive deficits to be a subclinical but abnormal state that presages dementia. Amnestic MCI, mild cognitive disorder, and mild neurocognitive disorder belong to the latter conceptualization. The occurrence of neuropsychiatric symptoms in MCI and the similarity of these symptoms to those of early AD suggest that these symptoms may assist in identifying patients in the earlier stages of AD and distinguishing them from patients with other disorders.

Acknowledgments

This study was supported by an Alzheimer's Disease Research Center grant (AG16570) from the National Institute on Aging, an Alzheimer's Disease Research Center of California grant, and the Sidell-Kagan Foundation.

References

1. Mendez MF, Martin RJ, Smyth KA, Whitehouse PJ. Psychiatric symptoms associated with Alzheimer's disease. J Neuropsychiatry Clin Neurosci 1990; 2:28–33.

2. Mega MS, Cummings JL, Fiorello T, Gornbein J. The spectrum of behavioral changes in Alzheimer's disease. Neurology 1996; 46:130–135.

3. Merriam AE, Aronson MK, Gaston P et al. The psychiatric symptoms of Alzheimer's disease. J Am Geriatr Soc 1988; 36:7–12.

4. Olin JT, Schneider LS, Katz IR et al. Provisional diagnostic criteria for depression of Alzheimer disease. Am J Geriatr Psychiatry 2002; 10:125–128.

5. Jeste DV, Finkel SI. Psychosis of Alzheimer's disease and related dementias. Diagnostic criteria for a distinct syndrome. Am J Geriatr Psychiatry 2000; 8:29–34.

6. Rabins PV, Mace NL, Lucas MJ. The impact of dementia on the family. JAMA 1982; 248:333–335.

7. Steele C, Rovner B, Chase GA, Folstein M. Psychiatric symptoms and nursing home placement of patients with Alzheimer's disease. Am J Psychiatry 1990; 147:1049–1051.

8. O'Donnell BF, Drachman DA, Barnes HJ et al. Incontinence and troublesome behaviors predict institutionalization in dementia. J Geriatr Psychiatry Neurol 1992; 5:45–52.

9. Kaufer DI. Cholinergic therapy for neuropsychiatric symptoms in neurologic disorders. Curr Psychiatry Rep 1999; 1:78–84.

10. Cummings JL. Cholinesterase inhibitors: a new class of psychotropic compounds. Am J Psychiatry 2000; 157:4–15.

11. Reisberg B, Franssen E, Sclan SG et al. Stage specific incidence of potentially remediable behavioral symptoms in aging and Alzheimer's disease: a study of 120 patients using the BEHAVE-AD. Bull Clin Neurosci 1989; 54:95–112.

12. Broe GA, Henderson AS, Creasey H et al. A case–control study of Alzheimer's disease in Australia. Neurology 1990; 40:1698–1707.

13. Li YS, Meyer JS, Thornby J. Longitudinal follow-up of depressive symptoms among normal versus cognitively impaired elderly. Int J Geriatr Psychiatry 2001; 16:718–727.

14. Stern Y, Mayeux R, Sano M et al. Predictors of disease course in patients with probable Alzheimer's disease. Neurology 1987; 37:1649–1653.

15. Drevets WC, Rubin EH. Psychotic symptoms and the longitudinal course of senile dementia of the Alzheimer type. Biol Psychiatry 1989; 25:39–48.

16. Petersen RC, Doody R, Kurz A et al. Current concepts in mild cognitive impairment. Arch Neurol 2001; 58:1985–1992.

17. Morris JC, Storandt M, Miller JP et al. Mild cognitive impairment represents early-stage Alzheimer disease. Arch Neurol 2001; 58:397–405.

18. Bischkopf J, Busse A, Angermeyer MC. Mild cognitive impairment—a review of prevalence, incidence and outcome according to current approaches. Acta Psychiatr Scand 2002; 106:403–414.

19. Tierney MC, Szalai JP, Snow WG et al. Prediction of probable Alzheimer's disease in memory-impaired patients: a prospective longitudinal study. Neurology 1996; 46:661–665.

20. Jack CR Jr, Petersen RC, Xu YC et al. Prediction of AD with MRI-based hippocampal volume in mild cognitive impairment. Neurology 1999; 52:1397–1403.

21. Kantarci K, Jack CR Jr, Xu YC et al. Mild cognitive impairment and Alzheimer disease: regional diffusivity of water. Radiology 2001; 219:101–107.

22. Catani M, Cherubini A, Howard R et al. (1)H-MR spectroscopy differentiates mild cognitive impairment from normal brain aging. Neuroreport 2001; 12:2315–2317.

23. Andreasen N, Minthon L, Vanmechelen E et al. Cerebrospinal fluid tau and Abeta42 as predictors of development of Alzheimer's disease in patients with mild cognitive impairment. Neurosci Lett 1999; 273:5–8.

24. Cummings JL, Mega M, Gray K et al. The Neuropsychiatric Inventory: comprehensive assessment of psychopathology in dementia. Neurology 1994; 44:2308–2314.

25. Jost BC, Grossberg GT. The evolution of psychiatric symptoms in Alzheimer's disease: a natural history study. J Am Geriatr Soc 1996; 44:1078–1081.

26. Rubin EH, Kinscherf DA. Psychopathology of very mild dementia of the Alzheimer type. Am J Psychiatry 1989; 146:1017–1021.

27. Wands K, Merskey H, Hachinski VC et al. A questionnaire investigation of anxiety and depression in early dementia. J Am Geriatr Soc 1990; 38:535–538.

28. Braak H, Braak E. Neuropathological stageing of Alzheimer-related changes. Acta Neuropathol (Berl) 1991; 82:239–259.

29. Morris JC, Price AL. Pathologic correlates of nondemented aging, mild cognitive impairment, and early-stage Alzheimer's disease. J Mol Neurosci 2001; 17:101–118.

30. Grober E, Dickson D, Sliwinski MJ et al. Memory and mental status correlates of modified Braak staging. Neurobiol Aging 1999; 20:573–579.

31. Petry S, Cummings JL, Hill MA, Shapira J. Personality alterations in dementia of the Alzheimer type. Arch Neurol 1988; 45:1187–1190.

32. Mega MS, Cummings JL. Frontal-subcortical circuits and neuropsychiatric disorders. J Neuropsychiatry Clin Neurosci 1994; 6:358–370.

33. Craig AH, Cummings JL, Fairbanks L et al. Cerebral blood flow correlates of apathy in Alzheimer disease. Arch Neurol 1996; 53:1116–1120.

34. Duffy JD, Campbell JJ 3rd. The regional prefrontal syndromes: a theoretical and clinical overview. J Neuropsychiatry Clin Neurosci 1994; 6:379–387.

35. Marin RS, Firinciogullari S, Biedrzycki RC. Group differences in the relationship between apathy and depression. J Nerv Ment Dis 1994; 182:235–239.

36. Rubin EH, Drevets WC, Burke WJ. The nature of psychotic symptoms in senile dementia of the Alzheimer type. J Geriatr Psychiatry Neurol 1988; 1:16–20.

37. Sultzer DL, Mahler ME, Mandelkern MA et al. The relationship between psychiatric symptoms and regional cortical metabolism in Alzheimer's disease. J Neuropsychiatry Clin Neurosci 1995; 7:476–484.

38. Mentis MJ, Weinstein EA, Horwitz B et al. Abnormal brain glucose metabolism in the delusional misidentification syndromes: a positron emission tomography study in Alzheimer disease. Biol Psychiatry 1995; 38:438–449.

39. Zubenko GS, Moossy J, Martinez AJ et al. Neuropathologic and neurochemical correlates of psychosis in primary dementia. Arch Neurol 1991; 48:619–624.

40. Farber NB, Rubin EH, Newcomer JW et al. Increased neocortical neurofibrillary tangle density in subjects with Alzheimer disease and psychosis. Arch Gen Psychiatry 2000; 57:1165–1173.

6

Cognitive rehabilitation in mild cognitive impairment and prodromal Alzheimer's disease

Martial Van der Linden, Anne-Claude Juillerat and Xavier Delbeuck

An increasing number of studies have demonstrated the efficacy and effectiveness of various cognitive interventions in persons with mild to moderate Alzheimer's disease (AD).[1,2] Because AD is characterized by a progression of neuropathologic damage, the cognitive interventions have to be continually adapted to changes in the patient's condition, and directly focused on daily-life situations, with the purpose of short-term effectiveness.[3,4] In addition, due to a reduction of processing resources as well as planning and comprehension difficulties frequently associated with AD, cognitive improvement (that is, the use of a facilitation strategy each time it is necessary; for example, using a face–name imagery mnemonic technique each time the patient has to learn a new name) will be very difficult for most AD patients. Indeed, the continual adoption of a facilitating technique by the patient is very demanding: it requires extensive practice to automate the use of a facilitating strategy, the acquisition of an appropriate belief system (which supports the strategy and corrects deleterious cognitive attitudes), and, finally, the ability to identify the specific daily-life situations in which the strategy is useful, to remember to use the strategy, and to maintain it in memory while it is applied.[5] Consequently, intervention in mild or moderate AD patients will mainly consist of temporarily facilitating cognitive processing on a particular occasion (for example, helping a patient to learn the neuropsychologist's name by indicating a mnemonic strategy), or teaching AD patients specific knowledge (skills or facts; for example, a particular name or route) to make them more autonomous in everyday life, by using techniques (such as spaced-retrieval, vanishing-cues, or errorless methods) that tap intact memory systems. Another option in AD patients' rehabilitation is to provide them with physical support or external aids (such as a memory book, diaries, and alarms) or to structure their (physical or human) environment to reduce the impact that cognitive deficits may have on everyday activities. Furthermore, the management of cognitive and behavioral problems in AD patients also implies the active participation of a caregiver.

The caregiver should be trained to adapt to the patient's physical environment, help with the use of external aids, and favor the use of optimizing factors and preserved capacities. The caregivers should also be trained to choose the best conditions for interactions with the patient (for example, not interacting in dual-task situations), to use differential reinforcement in order to change the maladaptive behaviors of the patient,[6] and to improve their competence in accompanying the patient in a way that should have a positive effect on the patient. Finally, a cognitive approach to rehabilitation of mild to moderate AD patients requires adapted structures, for both assessment and management. A promising approach seems to be the creation of day-care centers, in which a real-life environment can be reproduced, optimization strategies can be put in place, and satisfying leisure activities can be proposed.[1]

Besides mild and moderate AD patients, it has become recently apparent that another group of persons, those in the prodromal phase of AD, might also benefit from cognitive interventions.

Mild cognitive impairment and prodromal Alzheimer's disease

In recent years, a great deal of interest in dementia research has moved toward a transitional state between normal aging and mild AD.[7–9] Indeed, as publicity and awareness about the importance of AD increase, more and more elderly persons spontaneously present to their general practitioners or to memory clinics, asking for advice and help about cognitive difficulties. In addition, the increasing sophistication of diagnostic tools in dementia research has allowed identification of a group of elderly subjects with cognitive deficits who do not yet meet the criteria for dementia, but are at high risk of conversion. Various labels have been applied to this 'at-risk' group: mild cognitive impairment (MCI), aging-related cognitive decline (ARCD), cognitive impairment no dementia (CIND), questionable AD, minimal AD, prodromal AD, or clinical dementia rating (CDR)[10] grade 0.5. Recent evidence suggests that with time most patients will develop AD. For example, data from the Rochester study[7] shows that 80% of MCI subjects observed for more than 10 years have developed AD within a 6-year period. However, it should be noted that etiologic heterogeneity among persons with MCI could be more important than previously reported: for example, cerebrovascular disease seems to be underestimated as a potential cause of MCI.[11]

The importance of this 'at-risk' group is that they are considered to be an appropriate target for dementia-prevention strategies. Indeed, it has been suggested that these individuals should be identified because the objective of treatment is to intervene at the earliest possible stage of AD and to stop damage before any significant cognitive and functional decline has been observed. It has also been argued that informed knowledge of this predementia state may allow the patients to plan for their future while they still have the cognitive abilities to do so.

However, there is no evidence at present that MCI is amenable to treatment (but a number of clinical drug trials are being conducted in this population).[12] In addition, the clinical and neuropsychological criteria with which to best define the MCI group remain controversial.[9] For example, Ritchie et al[13] showed that criteria for MCI (that is, memory complaints insufficient to interfere with daily-life functioning, evidence of memory deficits on memory tests, and preservation of other cognitive abilities) applied to a general population had low sensitivity and predictability for dementia over 3 years. However, ARCD (defined by impairment in any of a wide range of cognitive functions, and not specifically memory) had greater predictive value in terms of conversion to AD, and was more stable over time than MCI. Also remaining to be developed is an efficient screening procedure that could be applied to the general population to identify with high predictability people with cognitive impairment who will develop dementia. In a recent study, Palmer et al[14] showed that a simple three-step procedure that simulates routine clinical practice (exploration of self-reported memory complaints, performance on a global cognitive test, and performance on specific neuropsychological tests) has a high predictive value for dementia at 3 years, but it identified only 18% of people in the preclinical phase (because of the low sensitivity of the measures). Finally, it should be mentioned that labeling persons with a disease might have significant adverse psychological and psychosocial consequences. Consequently, it is clear that clinicians should be very cautious in designating a patient as being in the prodromal phase of dementia. Moreover, differential management should be conceived for MCI patients discovered by applying research criteria, who may be unaware of their cognitive deficits (or attribute them to normal aging), and for those who present clinically, complaining about cognitive difficulties and asking for help.[7] In these 'clinically presented' individuals, it seems possible to propose cognitive interventions to lessen their functional disabilities and distress, even if the clinician finally decides not to make the diagnosis of preclinical dementia, after having considered the disadvantages of such a diagnosis as well as the uncertainties about the evolution of the condition. Furthermore, the cognitive interventions could also help to delay the (possible) appearance of more disabling cognitive and functional difficulties.

The objectives of the cognitive interventions in persons with MCI and prodromal AD might be relatively different from those conducted in mild and moderate AD patients. For example, cognitive improvement, rather than simple temporary facilitation, might be considered in some patients. Furthermore, as a number of persons with MCI and prodromal AD patients are still relatively autonomous, professionally active, and aware of their difficulties, the neuropsychologist will have to examine the impact of the deficits not only on the personal, familial, and social adjustments of the patients, but also on their professional integration. Finally, when the diagnosis of possible preclinical dementia is made, the patients may also be helped to understand the disease, learn how to deal wisely with it, and turn towards those goals in life that do not yet have to be given up. In addition, more general problems, such as the disease prognosis, the treatment perspectives, the financial and legal arrangements, or the biological inheritance, will also have to be addressed. Put differently, it clearly appears that more than ever, during the development of intervention in prodromal AD, one should consider that the patient is a responsible participant.

Before describing the cognitive rehabilitation strategies that could be adopted for MCI subjects and prodromal AD patients, it is necessary to describe more precisely the cognitive and functional deficits that are observed in these patients.

Neuropsychological characteristics of mild cognitive impairment and prodromal Alzheimer's disease

Episodic memory disorders have consistently been demonstrated in MCI and prodromal AD patients.[15–18] However, several studies have also found that there may be other types of cognitive dysfunction, especially executive deficits.[18–21] More recently, Copeland et al[22] demonstrated that changes in personality (such as irritability and passivity) are more common among persons in the prodromal phase of AD (those diagnosed with AD on follow-up) than among persons with memory changes who do not progress to meet clinical criteria for probable AD within the same follow-up period. Furthermore, mild depressive symptoms were also more common among persons in the prodromal phase of AD. Interestingly, symptoms of personality change, but not depressive symptoms, were related to the rate of progression of functional difficulties over time, specifically, those functional changes that were related to cognitive changes. The authors hypothesized that increased passivity in prodromal AD is related to increased cognitive decline: as the persons are overwhelmed by complex and demanding tasks, they become more passive as a result. Similarly, they also suggested that the symptoms of irritability might be related to the awareness of increased difficulties in daily functioning (a relation that may be lost as the disease progresses, along with reduced insight). However, according to Copeland et al,[22] it is also possible that prodromal irritability constitutes an early manifestation of psychotic symptoms (such as delusions which are frequently reported in patients with mild AD, especially the delusion that people are stealing things).[23] More specifically, persons in the prodromal phase of AD may be irritable about having misplaced something, but have sufficient memory to be aware of their own involvement in the episode. However, as the disease progresses, the patients may lose the ability to retrieve the contextual information of the episode; consequently, delusional thinking may develop.

A large number of studies have shown that the nature of the defective processes can vary considerably from one AD patient to another.[24] For example, striking evidence illustrating the heterogeneity of deficits in AD came from a study conducted by Galton et al,[25] in which the clinical and neuropsychological profile of 13 patients with pathologically proven AD was described. Four patients showed a typical neuropsychological pattern, with episodic memory deficits as the initial feature, and subsequent involvement of attentional, language, semantic memory, and visuospatial abilities. The other patients could be considered to be demonstrating an atypical profile, since their initial and major cognitive deficit did not affect episodic memory: six patients showed progressive (fluent and nonfluent) aphasia, one patient showed progressive visual dysfunction, and two patients showed progressive biparietal syndrome. There were no differences between the typical and atypical presentations with respect to age at presentation, length of illness, or the length of time that symptoms were reported before presentation at the memory clinic. By the time of neuropsychological assessment, most, but not all, of the typical and atypical patients showed evidence of a more global cognitive impairment. Although the majority of patients had deficits in episodic memory, two patients did not present such impairment. Thus, this study clearly demonstrated the large spectrum of AD presentations, but the way these various presentations progressively develop in the prodromal period remains unclear at present.

Nevertheless, Mapstone et al[26] recently showed that visuospatial impairment (impaired visual motion processing) might develop as an independent sign of degenerative disease, possibly preceding the clinical onset of AD. It should also be noted that a breakdown and extension of the MCI definition into three subtypes has been proposed by Petersen et al:[7] a purely amnesic syndrome, an impairment of a single memory domain of cognition, and a slight cognitive impairment in multiple domains of cognition. Finally, Geschwind et al[27] showed that nondemented individuals with known mutation carrier status for a highly penetrant, dominantly inherited dementing condition (frontotemporal dementia and parkinsonism linked to chromosome 17) showed evidence of cognitive dysfunction in the frontal/executive system, with unimpaired performance on several tasks assessing memory, language, and visuospatial abilities. These executive deficits were apparent in some of the youngest mutation carriers many decades prior to the predicted onset of dementia. In addition, the lack of correlation of the executive deficits with aging suggests that these impairments reflect the baseline functioning of these subjects. According to Geschwind et al,[27] these findings are consistent with a 'cognitive reserve' view[28] proposing that the baseline state of a particular brain region may influence its susceptibility to neurodegenerative processes. Put differently, due to developmental predisposition, the degenerative process would start in the most vulnerable brain regions (associated with less cognitive reserve) and later would involve more widespread areas of the brain. This developmental and 'cognitive resource' view seems to be consistent with the focal nature, at onset, of most neurodegenerative diseases.

One of the criteria for MCI is preservation of functional everyday abilities. This is an intriguing point if we consider that memory difficulties may be a very disabling disorder for a person who is still professionally active. In fact, Morris et al[29] and Tabert et al[30] showed that the interference of cognitive deficits with activities of daily living can be revealed by a detailed informant history in most subjects meeting the criteria of MCI, suggesting that, in fact, MCI represents early-stage AD (a view supported by the existence of neuropathologic features of AD). Similarly, Artero et al[31] also found that difficulties in the performance of everyday activities are more frequent in non-demented subjects with mild cognitive deficits than in the general population. In addition, this study showed that difficulties with visuospatial tasks have the greatest impact on ability to perform everyday activities, with loss of ability to use the telephone being the most useful indicator of the degree of underlying impairment. Furthermore, high premorbid levels (that is, high intelligence quotient and education) are seen to protect against activity loss.

More recently, Griffiths et al[32] assessed financial capacity in MCI patients, AD patients, and control subjects, using a standardized psychometric capacity measure (the Financial Capacity Instrument [FCI]). The FCI consists of 18 financial ability tests and nine domains of financial activity. The control and MCI groups performed significantly better than AD patients on most financial capacity measures. However, individuals with MCI showed significant, albeit mild, deficits in FCI domains of conceptual knowledge, cash transactions, bank statement management, bill payment, and overall financial capacity. It should be noted that impairment in overall financial capacity was not observed in all MCI participants. An interesting aspect of MCI patient performance on the FCI was a possible dissociation, in some tasks, of preserved financial knowledge and defective practical application of this knowledge, suggesting the contribution of executive dysfunction. Nevertheless, future research should attempt to investigate more directly the nature of the deficits affecting financial abilities in MCI patients.

It appears clearly from all these data that a better understanding of the impact of MCI and prodromal AD requires more reliable, sensitive, and specific assessment tasks to explore both functional abilities and deficits in various cognitive and affective domains.[9] Nevertheless, there is now some evidence that MCI and prodromal AD are associated with several types of cognitive, mood, personality, and functional difficulties, a condition which could be usefully addressed by specific cognitive interventions.

Cognitive interventions in mild cognitive impairment and prodromal Alzheimer's disease

Cognitive intervention in MCI or prodromal AD patients might be, at least partly, conceived in the light of the 'cognitive reserve' view,[28] which suggests that aspects of life experience supply a set of skills that allow an individual to cope with progressing AD pathology for a longer time before the degenerative process becomes clinically apparent. Therefore, one of the contributions of cognitive rehabilitation might be to provide a reserve that delays the onset of clinical manifestations, in relation to cognitive abilities not yet affected by the disease. In this regard, Scarneas et al[33] showed that engagement in leisure activities may reduce the risk of incident dementia: even when ethnic group, education, occupation, baseline cognitive performance, health limitations on social activities, cerebrovascular disease, and depression were controlled for, subjects with high leisure activity had 38% less risk of developing dementia, and this result has been replicated after eliminating subjects with borderline dementia (CDR = 0.5), which might lower leisure activity due to early disease. Even if the possibility that low leisure activity reflects early disease consequences cannot be entirely excluded, this study suggests that enhanced activity might reduce the risk of developing dementia. More recently, in a positron emission tomography study, Scarneas et al[34] observed that at any given level of clinical severity of AD, there is a greater degree of brain pathologic involvement in patients who have less engagement in social, intellectual, and physical activities, even when education and IQ are taken into account. These brain-imagery findings confirm that life experiences and activities may contribute to the ability to cope with the pathologic changes in AD, and they also indicate the possibility of interventions that might delay the onset of clinical symptoms of the disease.

Another objective of cognitive rehabilitation could be to improve defective cognitive performance, through the use of alternative (unaffected) cognitive processes (a reorganization strategy), by exploiting optimization factors (a facilitation strategy), or by providing the patients with external aids and structuring the environment to lessen the impact of cognitive deficits on everyday functioning. Finally, if certain personality changes (such as apathy) constitute (even partly) a reaction to the existence of a cognitive decline,[22] it might be hypothesized that decreasing the impact of the cognitive deficits will have a positive effect on personality. Thus, we recently showed that restoring a leisure activity (knitting), at home in a mild AD patient, by proposing several adaptations designed to minimize the impact of the cognitive impairments on knitting, significantly decreased the patient's apathy and depressive mood.[3]

Until now, very few studies have explored the efficacy of cognitive interventions in MCI and prodromal AD subjects. Nevertheless, some general principles guiding cognitive rehabilitation in these populations may be proposed. First, before implementing a rehabilitation program, it is crucial to understand the nature of the dysfunctions, and to identify the preserved abilities and optimization factors that could be exploited in the intervention. In addition, it is also necessary to identify the consequences of cognitive disorders in everyday activities. Indeed, the purpose of rehabilitation is not to increase performance on cognitive tests but to improve the quality of life for the patient and family caregivers. In this respect, the simulation of everyday cognitive activities is a particularly well-adapted approach. This simulation approach to assessment should allow the examiner to discern the nature of the impairments affecting everyday activities. However, this can only be done if a precise cognitive analysis of the processes involved in each activity is conducted according to existing theoretical models. Even if it is not sufficiently articulated on cognitive models and therefore does not really permit us to understand the nature of the observed deficits, the FCI, developed by Marson et al[35] and recently administered by Griffiths et al[32] to persons with MCI, constitutes a promising example of what might be an exploration of daily life activities.

Because memory impairments seem to be frequently observed in MCI and prodromal AD subjects, it is particularly important to determine the nature of these deficits, as well as their impact on everyday life, and to identify which form of cognitive support would improve memory performance in these persons. When considering the different ways of facilitating memory, it is crucial to characterize the specific memory problem. Does the person have to remember to do something (a prospective memory task) or rather to remember some facts or episodes? The aids usually involve helping the person to remember to do things by external memory aids (diaries, alarms, etc.). In cases where the situation concerns memory for facts or episodes, we must ask whether the problem lies at the encoding level (that is, how can one learn something in order to maximize later recall?), or at the retrieval phase (that is, how can one retrieve a piece of information believed to have entered memory?). If the problem is to acquire new information, the encoding strategy will be different, depending on whether the 'to-be-learned' material is organized and meaningful or not. In the case of meaningful information (for example, a text or a conference), the subject's task will be to increase comprehension of the material by relating the different pieces of information to each other, and by relating them to pre-existing knowledge (by using active learning, self-testing, etc.). In contrast, if the to-be-encoded material is poorly structured or meaningless, the person will have to impose meaning and relationships. For this latter purpose, one may resort to mnemonic techniques that will make up for the lack of meaning and supply retrieval cues. Finally, if the memory problem is located at the retrieval stage, relevant cues that elicit recall and whose relevance depends on the initial encoding situation will have to be found.

In this prospect, two recent studies[36,37] found that prose recall was significantly impaired in very mild AD patients (CDR = 0.5) and persons with MCI. Because this deficit is more dramatic for surface information recall than for reproduction of gist-based meaning information, Johnson et al[37] suggest that the difficulty seen in prose recall in very mild AD patients represents a deficit in the control of attention: put differently, they hypothesize that information fades more rapidly in these patients because the central executive component of working memory may be forced to engage in other demanding control tasks, such as verbally outputting the integrated information. This interpretation suggests that prose memory may be facilitated in prodromal

AD patients or persons with MCI by using 'refreshment' techniques, which should permit them to reactivate information continuously in working memory (for example, dividing text material into several parts, where each part is summarized before the presentation of the following part). As some degree of surface information processing is certainly necessary to formulate gist-based representations (even if several other factors are probably involved), an increased maintenance of surface information should improve recall of gist-related information. Gist recall may also be facilitated by using a method to organize material, to highlight the salient elements, and to increase the subject's interactions with the text, such as the PQRST (Preview; Question; Read; State; Test) method[38] or a technique leading the person to extract the different propositions from the text and reinsert them in a story schema.[39] Interestingly, Chapman et al[36] observed that while 13 of 20 subjects with MCI were impaired in a main idea-recall task (one of the three tasks given to evaluate gist-level processing), all MCI persons showed impaired recall of details, suggesting that in prodromal stages of AD, memory for details may precede gist-level deficits. However, as mentioned by the authors, it might be that MCI subjects with preserved gist-level discourse processing show a different conversion pattern (for example, being slower to convert or remaining nondemented). Finally, it should be noted that gist-preserved persons with MCI could be more responsive to some cognitive interventions (especially because they maintain higher levels of comprehension and inferential processing).

Recently, memory rehabilitation in mild or moderate AD patients has focused on teaching specific factual information by using techniques (such as the spaced-retrieval technique, which consists of prompting recall of information over increasingly longer retention intervals, or the vanishing-cues procedure, which involves giving subjects a gradually withdrawn cue) considered to exploit spared implicit memory abilities in AD. It has also been argued that both the spaced-retrieval and vanishing-cues techniques may have succeeded because an indirect result of these methods was to limit the opportunity for subjects to commit errors: indeed, according to Baddeley and Wilson,[40] patients with severe episodic memory deficits do not learn implicit memory tasks well when they are allowed to make errors during training, because they cannot remember and eliminate errors during the learning process. In fact, if the vanishing-cues and spaced-retrieval techniques are really based on implicit memory processes, it follows that they should not be necessarily beneficial to MCI or prodromal AD patients who show relatively mild episodic memory difficulties, because, in these patients, the exploitation of implicit memory will be contaminated by residual explicit memory ability. Nevertheless, it has been shown that the reduction of errors during motor-skill learning by normal subjects places less demand on explicit, attention-demanding resources than do skills acquired in an error-prone learning condition.[41] This reduced demand on attention after the adoption of an implicit learning process appears to confer insusceptibility to performance breakdown under distraction,[41] and robustness of performance under stress.[42] All these beneficial effects suggest that motor-skill learning without errors should be particularly recommended in MCI and prodromal AD patients.

Besides the exploration and rehabilitation of memory impairments, further studies are clearly needed to examine the nature of other cognitive deficits and to identify optimization factors in MCI and prodromal AD persons. In particular, a better understanding of executive deficits and their impact on everyday life constitutes an important challenge to both diagnosis and rehabilitation purposes. Recently, Miyake et al[43] found that three executive functions (shifting between mental sets or tasks, updating and monitoring of working memory contents, and inhibition of prepotent responses) are separable, but are also moderately correlated with one another, thus indicating both the unity and the diversity of executive functions. They also suggested that the simultaneous coordination of multiple tasks might be another distinct executive function. It is therefore possible that those executive deficits in MCI or prodromal AD are not global in nature, and that there is some specificity of impairment (along with specific impact on everyday activities). Even if the nature of executive deficits in MCI or prodromal AD patients remains to be determined, it is nevertheless possible to indicate several methods to rehabilitate executive functioning:[44,45] adapting the accomplishment of the everyday activities (for example, keeping instructions simple and unambiguous or suppressing irrelevant information); simplifying a complex task, teaching it as a routine, and organizing physical space (for example, using reminders of operating procedures or schedules to help with time management); training the selection and execution of cognitive plans (for example, planning scenarios or arranging errand-completion tasks to address planning, sequencing, initiation, and execution); and using self-instructional training (for example, verbalizing each step of a multistep task as it is completed).

Two studies have explored the effect of a multicomponent cognitive training program on memory functioning (and more general cognitive and behavioral functioning) in MCI subjects.[46,47] Belleville et al[46] administered to eight persons with MCI a training program devoted to improving episodic memory, working memory, and processing speed, as well as considering other aspects that could influence these cognitive abilities, such as a feeling of self-efficacy and stress. The results demonstrated a positive effect of the intervention on working and episodic memory tests, but not on processing speed. In addition, no improvement was observed on a task (verbal fluency) untargeted by the intervention, suggesting that the beneficial effects of the program could not be explained by a nonspecific influence. In a randomized clinical trial, Rapp et al[47] tested the efficacy of a cognitive and behavioral intervention to improve memory performance and attitudes towards memory in MCI participants. The program included education about memory loss and the factors that can influence memory performance (such as fatigue, anxiety, motivation, and appraised importance), relaxation training (systematic breathing), and memory-skills training (cueing, categorization, chunking, and method of loci). The trainers led group exercises using the trained skills, and assigned homework employing them. The treatment consisted of six, weekly group meetings lasting 2 hours each. Compared to a no-treatment control group, the treated participants had significantly better appraisals of their current and future memory abilities at the end of the intervention and at a 6-month follow-up. Concerning memory performance, there was only a tendency towards a better word-list recall in the trained group (but no real differences at post-test).

Both the studies of Belleville et al[46] and Rapp et al[47] revealed that it seems to be possible to improve some aspects of cognitive functioning as well as inadequate cognitive beliefs in persons with MCI. However, the effects of the training programs on quality of life and autonomy in everyday activities have not been specifically examined. Moreover, in Rapp et al's study,[47] no significant change was observed in the laboratory memory tasks after training. More generally, in both studies, the intervention programs have not been designed from a detailed analysis of the particular problems (or handicaps) revealed by each individual. Consequently, these global interventions might have very limited effects on quality of life. In addition, efficient memory functioning in everyday life seems to depend on the flexible use of different strategies adjusted to different memory situations. It follows from this that intervention programs should promote the adoption of multiple facilitation strategies. Considering the heterogeneity of the cognitive impairments, these strategies should be adapted to the particular deficits of each person (and also to his or her cognitive preferences). Consequently, rather than adopting ready-made programs, it seems to us more appropriate to design 'made-to-measure' interventions to address some concrete and specific daily-life difficulties of the patient, by taking into account both the nature of these difficulties and the existence of specific optimization factors. It should be noted that external cognitive aids (such as a memory book, diaries, alarms, etc.), as well as environmental adaptations designed to reduce the impact cognitive dysfunctions may have on everyday activities, have also to be 'made-to-measure' according to the person's difficulties, and, in some cases, a learning phase will have to be planned in order to teach the person how to use the method. Finally, as already mentioned, unlike most mild and moderate AD patients, a cognitive improvement may be considered in MCI or prodromal AD patients, but, in any case, this will require a relatively long and demanding acquisition and generalization phase. In this regard, spontaneous comments made by several participants in Rapp et al's study[47] indicated that they understood when to use the mnemonics, but they could not quickly and easily select or apply them. This suggests that participants may have needed more training sessions. One of us[48] recently observed that imagery mnemonics could be used to improve daily-life memory functioning in very early AD patients. More specifically, she showed that a 58-year-old man with very early AD (MMSE of 26) had spontaneously learned to use the face–name method, as well as the peg method (which consists of an imaged association of items to be memorized with a previously learned ordered list of peg words) every time he needs to acquire new names and short lists of errands.

In a prospective study, Ishizaki et al[49] have examined the effects of psychosocial interventions for elderly subjects with very mild AD (CDR = 0.5). The experimental group (14 subjects) participated in activities in a day-care-like setting once a week over a period of 6 months, whereas the control group (11 subjects) did not. The psychosocial program incorporated several classical intervention methods: reality orientation, reminiscence therapy, group therapy, and brief systemic therapy. The activities took place in a classroom-like setting and simple exercises, games, listening to music, singing, etc., were also included. Each group was re-evaluated after approximately 9 months. Immediately after the session, the experimental group showed a significant improvement of performance on a word-fluency task, a clinical global measure (Sum of Boxes in CDR, CDR-SB), and an observation scale assessing social interaction. However, unlike the experimental group, the control subjects showed a significant decline on the Mini-Mental State Examination (MMSE),[50] the digit span (forward and backward), and the Trail Making-A test. In addition, the experimental group revealed higher scores on the MMSE and the digit span than the control group at the 6-month follow-up. Finally, the same results were found after controlling for age, educational level, baseline cognitive performance, and affective status. These findings suggest that psychosocial intervention had beneficial effects for subjects with very mild AD.

However, more controlled studies are clearly required to identify the factors responsible for these benefits. In fact, the main limitations of these psychosocial interventions are that they are conducted without theoretical reference to the nature of the underlying deficits. Furthermore, they are based upon the implicit principle that all patients suffer from similar cognitive deficits and therefore will respond similarly to the same rehabilitation programs.[51] Nevertheless, MCI or prodromal AD patients are inclined to decrease their social activities because they are aware of their declining condition and the potential risky situations this may lead to. In this regard, proposing group activities that fit the patient's level of competence may help reduce the loss of confidence as well as depression, irritability, or apathy. It should be noted that the group activities could also supply a 'cognitive reserve' related to abilities, that are still preserved, allowing a delay in the onset of subsequent clinical manifestations. However, these psychosocial activities should be proposed after considering both the deficits and preserved abilities of each patient, and obviously their fields of interest.

Conclusion

An increasing number of studies suggest that MCI and prodromal AD patients suffer from various types of cognitive and affective deficits that begin to interfere with their everyday activities. Therefore, cognitive interventions should be made available to these persons to help them cope with their cognitive handicap. For the most part, the nature of these cognitive and functional difficulties has not yet been identified. A better understanding of these difficulties should allow us to develop more specific and efficient interventions. In addition, it also seems essential to determine whether and how cognitive and pharmacologic interventions may be combined to offer a more efficient treatment.

References

1. Van der Linden M, Juillerat AC, Adam S. Cognitive intervention. In: Mulligan R, Van der Linden M, Juillerat AC, eds. The Clinical Management of Early Alzheimer's Disease. Mahwah, NJ: Erlbaum, 2003:169–233.

2. Camp CJ, Foss JW. Designing ecologically valid memory interventions for persons with dementia. In: Payne DG, Conrad FG, eds. Intersections in Basic and Applied Memory Research. Mahwah, NJ: Erlbaum, 1997:311–325.

3. Adam S, Van der Linden M, Juillerat AC, Salmon E. The cognitive management of daily life activities in patients with mild to moderate Alzheimer's disease in a day care centre: a case report. Neuropsychol Rehab 2000; 10:485–509.

4. Clare L, Woods B. Editorial: a role for cognitive rehabilitation in dementia care. Neurospychol Rehab 2001; 11:193–196.

5. Camp CJ, McKitrick LA. Memory interventions in Alzheimer's-type dementia populations: methodological and theoretical issues. In: West RL, Sinnott JD, eds. Everyday Memory and Aging. Current Research and Methodology. New York: Springer-Verlag, 1992:155–172.

6. Bird, M. Psychosocial rehabilitation for problems arising from cognitive deficits in dementia. In: Hill RD, Bäckman L, Stigsdotter Neely A, eds. Cognitive rehabilitation in old age. Oxford: Oxford University Press, 2000:249–269.

7. Petersen RC, Doody R, Kurz A et al. Current concepts in mild cognitive impairment. Arch Neurol 2001; 58:1985–1992.

8. Burns A, Zaudig M. Mild cognitive impairment in older people. Lancet 2002; 360:1963–1965.

9. Thompson SA, Hodges JR. Mild cognitive impairment: a clinically useful but currently ill-defined concept? Neurocase 2002; 8:405–410.

10. Berg I. Clinical Dementia Rating (CDR). Psychopharmacol Bull 1988; 24:637–639.

11. DeCarli C. Mild cognitive impairment: prevalence, prognosis, aetiology, and treatment. Lancet 2003; 2:15–21.

12. Doraiswamy PM. Interventions in mild cognitive impairment and Alzheimer disease. Am J Geriatr Psychiatry 2003; 11:120–122.

13. Ritchie K, Artero S, Touchon J. Classification criteria for mild cognitive impairment: a population-based

validation study. Neurology 2001; 56:37–42.

14. Palmer K, Bäckman L, Winblad B, Fratiglioni L. Detection of Alzheimer's disease and dementia in the preclinical phase: population-based cohort study. BMJ 2003; 326:1–5.

15. Small BJ, Fratiglioni L, Vittanen M et al. The course of cognitive impairment in preclinical Alzheimer's disease: three- and 6-year follow-up of a population-based sample. Arch Neurol 2000; 57:839–844.

16. Elias MF, Beiser A, Wolf PhA et al. The preclinical phase of Alzheimer disease: a 22-year prospective study of the Framingham cohort. Arch Neurol 2000; 57:808–813.

17. Bäckman L, Small BJ, Fratiglioni L. Stability of the preclinical episodic memory deficit in Alzheimer's disease. Brain 2001; 124:96–102.

18. Crowell TA, Luis CA, Vanderploeg RD et al. Memory patterns and executive functioning in mild cognitive impairment and Alzheimer's disease. Aging Neuropsychol Cogn 2002; 9:288–297.

19. Fabrigoule C, Rouch I, Taberly A et al. Cognitive process in preclinical phase of dementia. Brain 1998; 121:135–141.

20. Albert MS, Moss MB, Tanzi R, Jones K. Preclinical prediction of AD using neuropsychological test. J Int Neuropsychol Soc 2001; 7:631–639.

21. Ready RE, Ot BR, Grace J, Cahn-Weiner DA. Apathy and executive dysfunction in mild cognitive impairment and Alzheimer disease. Am J Geriatr Psychiatry 2003; 11:222–228.

22. Copeland MP, Daly E, Hines V et al. Psychiatric symptomatology and prodromal Alzheimer's disease. Alzheimer Dis Assoc Disord 2003; 17:1–8.

23. Rubin E, Kinscherf D. Psychopathology of very mild dementia of the Alzheimer type. Am J Psychiatry 1989; 146:350–353.

24. Collette F, Van der Linden M, Juillerat AC, Meulemans T. Cognitive-neuropsychological aspects. In: Mulligan R, Van der Linden M, Juillerat AC, eds. The Clinical Management of Early Alzheimer's Disease. Mahwah, NJ: Erlbaum, 2003:35–73.

25. Galton CJ, Patterson K, Xuereb JH, Hodges JR. Atypical and typical presentations of Alzheimer's disease: a clinical, neuropsychological, neuroimaging and pathological study of 13 cases. Brain 2000; 123:484–498.

26. Mapstone M, Stefenella TM, Duffy CJ. A visuospatial variant of mild cognitive impairment: getting lost between aging and AD. Neurology 2003; 60:802–808.

27. Geschwind DH, Robidoux J, Alarcon M et al. Dementia and neurodevelopmental predisposition: cognitive dysfunction in presymptomatic subjects precedes dementia by decades in frontotemporal dementia. Arch Neurol 2001; 50:741–746.

28. Stern Y. What is cognitive reserve? Theory and research application of the reserve concept. J Int Neuropsychol Soc 2002; 8:448–460.

29. Morris JC, Storandt M, Miller JP et al. Mild cognitive impairment represents early-stage Alzheimer disease. Arch Neurol 2001; 58:397–405.

30. Tabert MH, Albert SM, Borukhova-Milov L et al. Functional deficits in patients with mild cognitive impairment: prediction of AD. Neurology 2002; 58:758–764.

31. Artero S, Touchon J, Ritchie K. Disability and mild cognitive impairment: longitudinal population-based study. Int J Geriatr Psychiatry 2001; 16:1092–1097.

32. Griffiths HR, Belue BS, Sicola BS et al. Impaired financial abilities in mild cognitive impairment. Neurology 2003; 60:449–457.

33. Scarmeas N, Levy G, Tang MX et al. Influence of leisure activity on the incidence of Alzheimer's disease. Neurology 2001; 57:2236–2242.

34. Scarmeas N, Zarahn E, Anderson KE et al. Association of life activities with cerebral blood flow in Alzheimer disease. Implications for the cognitive reserve hypothesis. Arch Neurol 2003; 60:359–365.

35. Marson DC, Sawrie SM, Snyder S et al. Assessing financial capacity in patients with Alzheimer's disease: a conceptual model and prototype instrument. Arch Neurol 2000; 57:877–884.

36. Chapman SB, Zientz J, Weiner M et al. Discourse changes in early Alzheimer disease, mild cognitive impairment, and normal aging. Alzheimer Dis Assoc Disord 2002; 16:177–186.

37. Johnson DK, Storandt M, Balota DA. Discourse analysis of logical memory recall in normal aging and in dementia of the Alzheimer type. Neuropsychology 2003; 17:82–92.

38. Glasgow RE, Zeiss RA, Barrera M Jr, Lewinshon PM. Case studies on remediating memory deficits in brain-injured patients. J Clin Psychol 1977; 33:1049–1054.

39. Van der Linden M, Van der Kaa MA. Reorganization therapy for memory impairments. In: Seron X, Deloche G, eds. Cognitive Approaches in Neuropsychological Rehabilitation. New York: Erlbaum, 1989: 105–158.

40. Baddeley AD, Wilson BA. When implicit learning fails: amnesia and the problem of error elimination. Neuropsychologia 1994; 32:53–68.

41. Maxwell JP, Masters RSW, Kerr E, Weedon E. The implicit benefits of learning without errors. Q J Exp Psychol 2001; 54:1049–1068.

42. Hardy L, Mullen R, Jones G. Knowledge and conscious control of motor actions under stress. Br J Psychol 1996; 87:621–636.

43. Miyake A, Friedman NP, Emerson MJ et al. The unity and diversity of executive functions and their contributions to complex 'frontal lobe' tasks: a latent variable analysis. Cogn Psychol 2000; 41:49–100.

44. Van der Linden M, Seron X, Coyette F. La prise en charge des troubles exécutifs [Rehabilitation of executive deficits]. In: Seron X, van der Linden M, eds. Traité de neuropsychologie clinique, vol. 2. Marseille: Solal, 2000:253–268.

45. Sohlberg MM, Mateer CA. Cognitive Rehabilitation: An Integrative Neuropsychological Approach. New York: Guilford Press, 2001.

46. Belleville S, Gilbert B, Gagnon ML et al. Intervention cognitive chez les personnes âgées souffrant d'un léger trouble de la cognition [Mild cognitive impairment]. Rev Med Brux 2002; 23(Suppl 1):A170 (Abstract).

47. Rapp S, Brenes G, Marsh AP. Memory enhancement training for older adults with mild cognitive impairment: a preliminary study. Aging Ment Health 2002; 6:5–11.

48. Juillerat AC. Utilisation d'une stratégie d'imagerie et d'un agenda électronique dans la prise en charge d'un patient présentant une maladie d'Alzheimer à un stade débutant, submitted.

49. Ishizaki J, Meguro K, Ohe K et al. Therapeutic psychosocial intervention for elderly subjects with very mild Alzheimer disease in a community: the Tajiri Project. Alzheimer Dis Assoc Disord 2002; 16:261–269.

50. Folstein MF, Folstein SE, McHugh RH. 'Mini-Mental State': a practical method for grading the cognitive state of patients for the clinician. J Psychiatr Res 1975; 12:189–198.

51. Van der Linden M, Seron X. Prise en charge des déficits cognitifs [Cognitive interventions]. In: Guard O, Michel B, eds. La maladie d'Alzheimer. Paris: Medsi/McGraw-Hill, 1989: 289–303.

7

Clinical trials design in the age of dementia treatments: Challenges and opportunities

Erich Mohr, C Lynn Barclay, Roberta Anderson and
John Constant

Introduction

The successful introduction of efficacious, nontoxic treatment options for
Alzheimer's disease (AD)[1–7] in most of the world has transformed both the
design and execution of clinical trials for antidementia agents. The availability of these compounds, although variable and not universal, has significantly
changed patient characteristics and availability for this kind of research.[8] In
addition to the target population and its definition, the question of the use of
placebo-controlled trial designs, the involvement of treated reference groups,
and the intended mode of treatment (symptomatic versus disease-modifying), as well as the emergence of surrogate markers, will all play a key role
on a go-forward basis.

The relative lack of availability of treatment-naive populations poses further
challenges in that patients who were treatment failures on currently available
cholinesterase inhibitors may form the basis of scientific conclusions in clinical
trials of new antidementia agents. In part to avoid the potential bias associated
with reliance on treatment failures and to utilize additional sources of patients,
trials increasingly include countries outside North America and Western Europe.
The conduct of these trials on a truly global basis requires close attention to
comparability of test materials, administration, and scoring in linguistically and
culturally diverse environments and divergent medical practices. The following
text provides an overview of these issues and suggests possible solutions. In a
highly dynamic field, these topics will continue to evolve rapidly, but many of the
fundamental principles will continue to apply in the future.

Definition of clinical trials population

While a number of approved compounds have been studied in potentially prodromic disease states[9,10] or in those with moderate to severe

disease,[11] the current research focus remains on mild to moderate stages AD.

The selection of AD patients on the basis of accepted criteria continues to be a core requirement of current regulatory submissions. However, even accepted benchmarks, such as the NINCDS–ADRDA[12] criteria, have recently come under scrutiny with respect to sensitivity and specificity. While sensitivity of these criteria has been reported as very high, relative specificity may be more variable, with figures in the literature as low as 0.23.[13] Nevertheless, while patients can vary significantly in terms of onset, clinical presentation, and disease course,[14,15] clinical diagnostic parameters in the hands of experienced clinicians tend to show sensitivity and specificity rates of approximately 90% or more, particularly in the more recent past.[16]

With time frames for trials typically in the 6-month range for symptomatic therapies, patient populations are needed which have the potential to show sufficient change in the untreated state within this time. The stipulation, then, of mild to moderate probable AD according to the NINCDS–ADRDA criteria[12] with evidence of current mental function between a low of 10–14 and a high of 24–26 on the Mini-Mental State Examination (MMSE),[17] as has commonly been done in the past, continues to be warranted. More controversial has been the recent proposal to limit participants to those who also have an ADAS-Cog score of ≥ 15, the concept being that only patients in this category will be able to show improvement toward the normal range of 0–10.[18]

The choice of relatively healthy subjects remains a sine qua non in dementia research in the early phases of drug development. Therefore, typical protocols require exclusion of most clinically significant illnesses. With respect to systemic conditions, this includes clinically significant pulmonary and cardiovascular disease within the last 6 months, such as chronic obstructive pulmonary disease, myocardial infarction, angina, and cardiac failure, or vital signs consistently outside acceptable ranges. Patients also typically excluded are those with significant hepatic and/or renal disease, insulin-dependent diabetes, or cancer within 5 years prior to baseline. These restrictions continue to be utilized to ensure no undue exposure of systemically weakened individuals prior to a full understanding of potential risks and efficacy.

Exclusion of any other cause of dementia or documented history of alcohol and/or drug abuse is also necessary to ensure, as much as possible, that the deficits detected on outcome measures are solely related to Alzheimer's pathology. Neurologic conditions which could affect cognition, including dementia following open-heart surgery, cardiac arrest, or significant head injury, must also be excluded. While it is generally not difficult to exclude Parkinson's disease, normal-pressure hydrocephalus, and seizure disorders, the differentiation of AD from diffuse Lewy body disease, or vascular or mixed dementia may not always be straightforward. Patients with vascular and mixed dementia are excluded, as much as possible, on the basis of history or physical findings of stroke or by the presence of infarct(s) on imaging procedures. While the latter criteria would not necessarily lead to the exclusion of a patient with widespread subcortical ischemic white-matter disease (periventricular leukomalcia) in the absence of clinical strokes, these exclusions will at least limit the contamination of the study population by patients who have a component of vascular dementia. Such a limitation is probably not feasible in patients with diffuse Lewy body disease. A recent investigation reported Alzheimer's pathology in 81% of cases with Lewy body dementia and Lewy body pathology in 93% of cases with the clinical diagnosis of AD.[19] Therefore, even though imaging parameters,[20–22] putative biological markers,[23–25] and biochemical indices (B_{12} and thyroid indices)[26] may all supply additional evidence with respect to the diagnosis of AD, ultimate disease classification continues to rest firmly on clinical grounds.[16,27,28]

A further potential confounding factor, generally having received less investigative attention, is psychiatric illness, either as a comorbid condition or as a misclassification of dementia.[29] In particular, depression may be a confounding factor, since memory disorders associated with depression, particularly in the episodic realm (memory dated in time and place), can be a significant part of the perception and expression of dementia.[30] Depressive illness is therefore a common cause of misdiagnosis and frequently coexists with dementia.[31] Likewise the presence of psychosis, potentially also present as a comorbid factor, particularly in the moderate stages of dementia, needs to be carefully ruled out, since its variable presence throughout a trial may significantly affect cognitive and other outcome measures. While actual diagnostic misclassification in this context is uncommon, caution needs to be exercised, since concomitant medication that may affect cognition must be disallowed at study entry or kept stable during the course of a trial. Patients may not, therefore, be able to receive maximally effective antidepressants or other psychotropics, which they would otherwise require, during a clinical trial.[32]

In addition to systemic, neurologic, and psychiatric patient evaluation, neuropsychological profiling continues to be of core importance. In order to exclude other diagnostic parameters and to provide a baseline for outcome measures in clinical trials, the purpose of neuropsychological testing typically includes screening for cognitive dysfunction, comprehensive neuropsychological assessment for early and/or complicated disease, evaluation of disease stage and progression, and, as part of this process, assessment of outcome of experimental therapeutic intercession.[30] Domains typically assessed are listed in Table 7.1.

Table 7.1. Diagnostic assessment for dementia: neuropsychological domains.

	Neuropsychological domains
(1)	Level of consciousness and attention
(2)	Orientation
(3)	Mood and motivation
(4)	Language
(5)	Memory
(6)	Praxis
(7)	Gnosia
(8)	Visuospatial and constructional tasks
(9)	Calculation
(10)	Abstraction
(11)	Judgment

Reprinted with permission of Martin Dunitz.[30]

Outcome measures

AD is a multifaceted disorder which affects cognition, psychiatric status, activities of daily living, quality of life, and caregiver burden, and it also has a substantial health-economic impact. Each of these facets can be measured. However, cognition and global functioning have traditionally been the primary areas of examination. The current research focus on mild to moderate disease is driven by two considerations:

1) Efficacy is typically accepted by evidence of a clinically meaningful and statistically significant change on a cognitive outcome measure and on a clinical global rating scale.
2) In order for us to be able to measure change on these instruments, patients must be sufficiently impaired at baseline to evidence a potential for change.

Cognitive outcome measures

The AD Assessment Scale, Cognitive Subscale[33] (ADAS-Cog) is currently the most widely used cognitive measure for assessing the efficacy of AD drug treatments. This test has high interrater and test–retest reliability, and is available in 10 equivalent English versions[33] to allow for repeated administration while minimizing practice effects. Experience with cholinesterase inhibitors shows that an effect size of 3 points on the ADAS-Cog relative to placebo over the course of 6 months yields a clinically meaningful result.[3] Of course, patients' ability to benefit from these treatments is influenced in part by their relative scores at baseline and their overall disease severity at that point.[34]

The rate of decline in AD patients generally follows a sigmoidal curve, with slow deterioration in the early stages of the illness, advancing to more rapid decline in the middle stages, and again slowing in the more advanced stages.[35–37] Specifically, earlier work has shown that individuals with ADAS-Cog scores of approximately 35 will lose in the vicinity of 12 ADAS-Cog points per year, while those with relatively mild scores (such as 15) or more severe ones (such as 60) will evidence deterioration across the span of a year at less than half the rate of the middle group (at approximately 5 points)[35] (Figure 7.1).

Therefore, inclusion of patients scoring beyond the very mild stages of the illness at study entry will substantially increase the chance to detect a treatment effect across the commonly employed 6-month trial length (see Figure 7.1[38]). However, at the severe end of the spectrum, in addition to the much slower deterioration curves,[35] the issue of test validity and reliability also plays a role. Specifically, alternative measures to the ADAS-Cog need to be considered, since patients in this stage of the illness are no longer testable on this instrument. Alternatives such as the Severe Impairment Battery[39] have been used successfully and reported in the literature.[11]

Global outcome measures

Global outcome measures are included in clinical trials of AD in order to help understand the overall clinical meaningfulness of an intervention in a patient's condition. The Clinician's Interview-Based Impression of Change (CIBIC-plus)[40] is the best-known global instrument and includes interviews of both

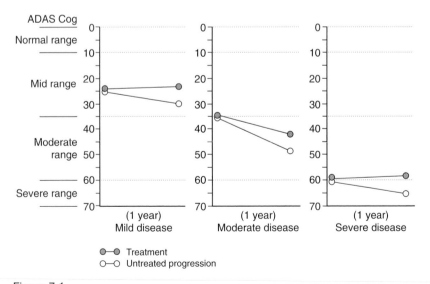

Figure 7.1

Schematic deterioration of untreated Alzheimer's disease patients in different disease stages across a 1-year time span, with average gains on cholinesterase inhibitors indicated.[34,38]

the patient and a caregiver. It is a 7-point scale and has been the most commonly used global measure in AD trials to date. It generally shows a 0.2–0.5 point change over the course of 6 months.[34] It has evolved over time,[41] the AD Cooperative Study–Clinical Global Impression of Change (ADCS–CGIC) being the most recent version.[40] It has reasonable validity and reliability up to 12 months.[40] However, the Clinical Dementia Rating (CDR),[42] a more structured interview for which extensive validity and reliability data are available,[41,43–50] may offer an advantage in long-term trials. The CDR has been validated over longer periods of time,[51] and, unlike the ADCS–CGIC, clear guidelines exist for its administration and scoring.[47,50] These guidelines will mitigate the negative impact of rater change, an unfortunate accompaniment of long-term trials. The CDR can be scored in two ways. A global score (0–3) can be allocated by synthesizing the individual scores from the six domains tested,[50] or a 'sum of boxes' score may be given by adding scores from the individual domains. The latter, by allowing for finer gradations in scoring, may provide more sensitivity to detect change. This, combined with the long-term data on its validity, has led to recommendations that the CDR sum of boxes be included as the global measure in AD trials lasting 12–24 months.[51]

There are further advantages to the CDR, especially in culturally and linguistically diverse patient populations. It is available in 17 languages, and a comprehensive, free Web-based tutorial is available through the AD Research Center (www.Alzheimer.wustl.edu/ardc2/Education). These substantial advantages all support the use of the CDR, rather than the ADCS–CGIC, in long-term trials in AD.

Other outcome measures

In addition to positive effects on cognition, demonstration of benefit on functional measures, such as those assessing activities of daily living, has been mandated by European regulatory authorities.[52] The Disability Assessment in Dementia (DAD) is a particularly good instrument to serve this function.[53] It has established validity and reliability (initial studies were done in English and French) and is currently available in several languages.[53] It measures both basic and instrumental activities of daily living and avoids some cultural and gender bias by scoring patients only on tasks which were part of their normal repertoire prior to the development of dementia. The DAD also has a consistent rate of decline over the course of 12 months in placebo-treated patients with mild to moderate AD,[54] and this is of particular relevance for the longer trials which will be needed to demonstrate disease modification.

Neuropsychiatric disturbances are an integral part of the clinical picture of AD and, though it is not required by regulatory authorities, all clinical trials of new therapeutic interventions in AD should include an instrument to assess these disturbances. The Neuropsychiatric Inventory (NPI)[55] and the Behavioral Pathology in AD scales (BEHAVE-AD)[56] have seen widespread use for this function. While both are valid and reliable,[55,56] the NPI may be the preferred option. It assesses a slightly broader scope of behavioral disturbances, valid, reliable versions are available in several languages, and it also includes a component which assesses the distress such behaviors cause to caregivers. Since caregiver distress due to neuropsychiatric symptoms is a significant cause of institutionalization, this is a particularly important outcome measure to collect.[57–59]

Other scales which measure individual behavioral symptoms, such as depression, do not sufficiently examine the spectrum of psychiatric pathology associated with AD and should not have a routine place in clinical trials of this disorder. The major role of such instruments is at screening, to exclude patients with major depression. Only scales which have been validated in demented patients are appropriate for inclusion. The Cornell Scale for Depression in Dementia, which involves independent interviews with the patient and caregiver, is an example of an instrument which meets this criterion.[60] While the Geriatric Depression Rating Scale has been validated in patients with MMSE scores as low as 14, its exclusive reliance on patient self-reporting may make it less useful, particularly with more advanced patients.[61,62]

Pharmacoeconomic measures are also gaining importance as an increasing incidence of dementia due to an aging population puts added burden on the health-care systems of the developed world. The number needed to treat (NNT)[63] to prevent a case of AD or to prevent one patient from requiring institutionalization is a measure which can probably be translated into monetary terms in many jurisdictions. However, since health-care systems, standards of practice, rates of institutionalization, and the bearer of the cost of various aspects of health care vary widely in different countries, across-the-board recommendations on pharmacoeconomic outcome measures are not possible. Interested readers are referred to Wimo et al for a comprehensive review of this topic.[64]

The special challenge of linguistically diverse global trials in Alzheimer's disease

The relatively large number of patients that will be required for trials of disease-modifying therapies and the continuing need to find treatment-naive patients for some trials of symptomatic agents (such as proof-of-concept or dose-finding studies) will result in a greater need to enroll patients from more diverse countries and linguistic backgrounds than has been the case to date. This will result in cross-cultural and linguistic challenges which will need to be addressed and overcome.

Cross-cultural outcome measures

The ADAS-Cog has been translated and validated in a number of different languages by EUROHARPID, Consortium to Establish a Registry for

AD (CERAD),[65] Grupo NORMACODEM,[66] Groupe de Reflexion sur les Évaluations Cognitives (GRECO), Beltz Test, and others. These organizations, however, have generally worked independently of one another, and the resulting translations are not necessarily uniform or equivalent. Moreover, several points of contact must be made to obtain permission to reproduce the various ADAS-Cog tests, and all relevant sections or equivalent versions may not be available in all required languages. Thus, additional translations and back translations may be required for each new global AD trial and must, in turn, be reviewed by a cross-cultural expert for face validity, general appropriateness, cultural fairness and relevance, and linguistic equivalence. Likewise, the use of abbreviated, edited, or modified versions of the various AD outcome measures still occurs frequently, potentially affecting the integrity and generalizability of results. In sum, relatively modest progress has been made on harmonizing translation efforts for outcome measures used in global AD clinical trials over the past 10 years.

In the absence of explicit regulatory guidelines on test translation and validation, a scientifically rigorous, streamlined, and economical approach to multilingual test development obliges the test developer to maintain version control in all languages. The test developer must be involved in providing translation specifications (to ensure linguistic equivalence of all items) and, subsequently, in the test validation and publication. With this approach, only a single point of contact is required to obtain the rights to reproduce the most current validated version of the required test in the desired languages. One example of a well-controlled test is the NPI,[55] which is available in 12 languages and can be reproduced only with permission of the author.

Importance of rater qualification and training

Reproducing various linguistically and culturally equivalent outcome measures is only the first step in ensuring global AD trial success. Rater qualification, experience, and trial-specific training are paramount in minimizing rater-error variance and optimizing interrater reliability. Rater qualifications and experience must be reviewed and approved prior to conducting any trial-specific testing to ensure that only individuals with appropriate backgrounds are permitted to perform assessments. Additionally, an intensive trial-specific rater training session on standard administration and scoring procedures must be provided, preferably in the local language, to ensure the integrity of the data and the accuracy of the results. Multimedia raters' workshops, including patient videotapes and scoring exercises using the audience-response keypad system, are highly effective for training raters.[67] Additionally, ongoing training sessions (meeting, Web-based, or telephone) should also be available for the duration of the clinical trial to accommodate any new raters.

Centralized scoring of subjective neuropsychological tests

In spite of comprehensive training of qualified raters, rater variability and error may potentially compromise the validity of the results and thereby jeopardize the success of the trial. Typical rater errors include those of incorrect scoring, arithmetic, transcription, and age calculation, the so-called clerical errors. One report on this subject noted that nearly 90% of raters made at least one clerical error in an investigation of 200 intelligence test results.[67] Since even qualified, well-trained raters make scoring errors on objective tests that purport to offer good interrater reliability and easy administration and scoring, the rate of error commission does not decrease with rater practice. Alternate methods of obtaining these scores should be sought where feasible.

Expert centralized scoring of neuropsychological tests is one potential option to address this issue. It is a cost-effective way to minimize rater error and ensure that no regional administration, scoring, or monitoring discrepancies occur. Centralized scoring may therefore significantly improve the accuracy of the data collected in global AD clinical trials. Where centralized scoring is not possible, careful attention to design of data collection forms may decrease some types of errors. For example, transcription and addition errors can be avoided by having raters fill out individual test items directly on the data-collection forms, rather than transcribing item scores or providing a simple summary score for the entire measure.

Reference groups in new trial designs

The design of clinical trials of antidementia agents in an age of the availability of efficacious treatment alternatives will need to incorporate the concept of equipoise, the relative balance of knowledge about new therapies being investigated versus those already in the physician's repertoire.[69] Alternatives to hitherto accepted placebo-controlled designs will need to be explored, since future designs, particularly in the area of disease modification, will probably require lengthy time periods, well beyond the 6 months currently considered standard.[8] The acceptability of placebo studies in untreated patients has been diminishing as increasing numbers of agents reach approval. For proof-of-concept studies, placebo control, especially in untreated patients, continues to be the preferred approach. Because of the short duration of exposure (12 weeks), it still is possible to conduct such trials. However, studies of longer duration are much more difficult. Six-month studies are probably the maximum duration that is feasible, but, in the absence of open-label extension studies, recruitment for these trials will remain difficult. Use of active controls and studying agents as add-on therapies in patients on stable doses of cholinesterase inhibitors are likely to become more common. This inclusion of cholinesterase inhibitors in all treatment arms, with placebo and active treatment being added to the appropriate arms, may become the new standard.

Trial design in mild to moderate Alzheimer's disease

Trial design for symptomatic therapies for AD has been well established and widely accepted. Regulatory agencies in Europe and North America have provided clear guidelines detailing the necessary features for such trials to result in marketing approval for a new therapeutic agent.

The US Food and Drug Administration (FDA) requires evidence that a treatment improves both cognition and global functioning in double-blind, placebo-controlled trials of sufficient duration to demonstrate meaningful benefit.[70] The European authorities[52] have added two additional requirements—a responder analysis and the need to show benefit on a functional measure such as activities of daily living. While behavioral endpoints have also been identified as important outcomes, the absolute requirement for statistical significance on such a measure has not been mandated.

These regulatory guidelines have led to a fairly standard approach to trial design for symptomatic therapies. Short-term studies (12 weeks) are typically used for proof-of-concept and dose-finding, but longer trials (6 months) are the standard for pivotal trials. Standard outcome measures include those of cognition, global functioning, activities of daily living, and behavioral symptoms. While not mandated by regulatory authorities, the advisability of including measures of caregiver burden, quality of life, and pharmacoeconomics has been increasingly recognized.

Studies of potentially disease-modifying agents

New therapeutic interventions are being developed which have the potential to modify underlying disease processes, and these present substantial challenges in trial design. Currently, for disease modification, no agent has been approved in any jurisdiction, no guidance has been issued by any regulatory agency, and no consensus on design exists among academics. Since no approved, validated, direct measures of disease progression currently exist, it is necessary to infer the presence of disease modification from measurement of standard clinical outcomes. Designs other than the traditional one of parallel-groups therefore required.

Five suggested designs for disease modification have been discussed in the literature to date, and all are two-period studies.[70–74] Two of them, the withdrawal design (WD) and the delayed or staggered start design, have received the most attention. The other three are variants of these designs. Because of the large patient numbers and the longer duration required for these trials, it will not be possible to recruit only treatment-naive patients for such studies. Instead, patients on stable doses of symptomatic therapy will have to be allowed entry.

Withdrawal designs

The WD, is a two-arm, two-period study (see Figure 7.2). In the first period, patients are randomized to active drug or placebo. In the second period, patients on active therapy are switched to placebo. Conceptually, if the benefit of the therapy was solely symptomatic, after a reasonable period of withdrawal the active group would become indistinguishable from the placebo group. If a disease-modifying effect is present, the active group will continue to be superior to placebo at the completion of period 2.

Although, theoretically this is a viable approach, from a practical standpoint, there are issues which limit the usefulness of this design. If an intervention has no symptomatic effect and does not actually reverse the disease to improve outcome scores, the difference between the groups must be driven solely by the deterioration in the placebo group. Historical information from trials before the era of approval of cholinesterase inhibitors suggests that the expected deterioration over 1 year in untreated patients on placebo in clinical trials is in the range of 5–7 points on the ADAS-Cog.[75,76] More recent clinical trial experience (unpublished data), suggests a smaller difference (2.5–4 points). This is not unexpected, given that, in the age of cholinesterase inhibitors, both caregivers and physicians are uncomfortable in entering patients with more moderate disease in placebo-controlled stud-

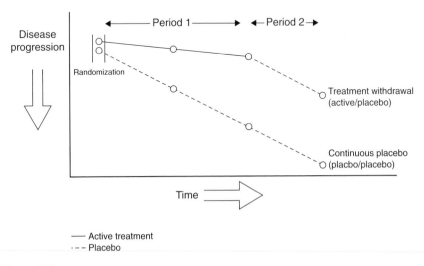

Figure 7.2
Withdrawal design.

ies where symptomatic treatment is not permitted. Patients with milder disease are therefore recruited, and these tend to experience a smaller decline in ADAS-Cog over the course of 1 year.[37] When disease-modifying treatments are being studied, it is also preferable to use a milder population, since these patients are more likely to achieve benefit. These latter numbers could, therefore, be anticipated in future trials.

From a clinical perspective, a slowing of progression by one-third is probably meaningful, but this would translate, in a year-long study of mild patients, to a difference between groups of only about 1–2 points on the ADAS-Cog. A 1-point difference on an ADAS-Cog is unlikely to be associated with a clinically meaningful change in the global measure; therefore, trials of longer than 1 year will be necessary. For longer studies, both higher dropout rates and higher variability in outcome measures can be expected.[73] This leads to the need to recruit larger numbers of patients or to extend the duration of period 1 beyond 1 year (see Table 7.2).

There are other practical and statistical issues which interfere with the utility of this design. While all patients will maintain their symptomatic therapy, because all patients will receive placebo at some point during the trial, it may be more difficult to recruit willing participants. Given the long nature of the study and the inevitability of patient deterioration, we can also expect that some patients (or caregivers) may insist on changing a patient's symptomatic therapy to try to maximize their symptom control. This must be avoided to protect the integrity of the trial results.

In year-long studies of symptomatic agents, dropouts in the order of 25–30%[77–79] are common and, in a withdrawal design, further dropouts could be expected in period 2, due to the lack of treatment. From a statistical perspective, the handling of dropouts is always problematic in a two-period design. In an intent-to-treat analysis, imputation of missing data may introduce bias, and data cannot be carried forward from period 1 to period 2. The alternative approach, analysis of observed cases only, introduces selection biases. In addition, it loses valuable data, and it will decrease the number of patients available for complete analysis.

Table 7.2. Sample size calculations for disease modification trials.

Difference in change in ADAS-Cog-score between groups	Number of subjects per group		
	12 Months*	18 Months**	24 Months***
1.5	932	1076	1165
2.0	526	607	657
2.5	338	390	422
3.0	235	271	294

Powered only to detect a difference in change in ADAS-Cog between groups. These numbers apply to all two- and three-arm studies discussed here. *Assuming 25% dropout; **assuming 35% dropout; ***assuming 40% dropout.

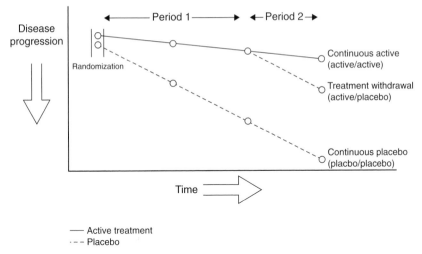

Figure 7.3
Randomized withdrawal design.

A further issue of concern in this design is that blinding of raters will be lost in the second period. Given the FDA's requirement of double-blind studies, it is unclear whether information from this period, information critical in separating symptomatic from disease-modifying effects, would be acceptable for making a labeling claim. A modification of the withdrawal design, the randomized withdrawal design, avoids unblinding by adding one additional arm to the study—a group which will continue active therapy throughout both periods (Figure 7.3). This makes it possible to differentiate disease-modifying from symptomatic effects with blinded data, at the cost of an increase in sample size. This increase in sample size does not result in a concomitant increase in power to differentiate symptomatic from disease-modifying effects.[74] Although this design is inefficient in this respect, recruitment would be facilitated since patients would be more likely to be exposed to active treatment than in the withdrawal design.

Delayed-start designs

In period 1 of the two-arm, delayed-start design, patients begin either active treatment or placebo. After a reasonable period of time (one sufficient to demonstrate disease modification), those who started on placebo are switched to active therapy (period 2) (see Figure 7.4). While this period is generally shorter than period 1, it must be of sufficient duration to show a symptomatic effect, should one be present. Practically speaking, because of the nature of the interventions that will employ this design, which would

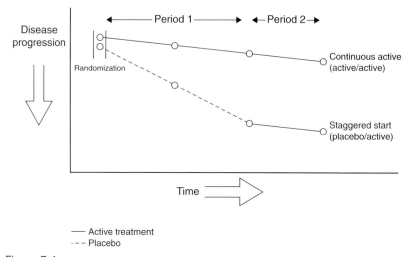

Figure 7.4

Delayed-start design.

include ones with a presumed delay in onset of benefit, it will probably not be possible to choose a duration less than 6 months for period 2.

It is presumed that in period 2, for an agent with symptomatic effects only, the outcomes of those who were initially randomized to placebo would converge on the results in the group initially randomized to active therapy. If the compound possessed disease-modifying capability, while the slope of the deterioration line for the placebo group would change, this line would not converge on the one of the group which received active treatment throughout.

Many of the same concerns exist with this design as with the withdrawal design. Large patient numbers will be required in the case of patients with mild AD, and handling of dropouts is problematic. In addition, double blinding will not be maintained in period 2 and could affect the integrity of the results. As with the withdrawal design, there is a variant of this design, the randomized delayed start, which, by incorporating an additional arm which remains on placebo for the duration of the trial, allows maintenance of the blinding (Figure 7.5). While this design requires more patients, who again do not contribute to an increase in power, it allows the differentiation of disease-modifying from symptomatic effects with blinded data.

The delayed-start design (but not the randomized delayed start) is one which would be much easier to convince patients and caregivers to participate in than the withdrawal design, since all patients can be guaranteed to receive active therapy. But it is probably not the preferred approach for several reasons. Both the delayed-start and the withdrawal designs require the same duration for period 1. However, the delayed-start design requires a

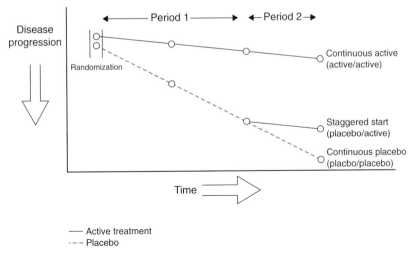

Figure 7.5
Randomized delayed-start design.

longer period 2. In the withdrawal design, period 2 must be sufficiently prolonged that any biological activity of the active drug is gone. Three months
is probably adequate for most agents. For the delayed-start design, because
it is likely that clinical effects will take time to become measurable, 6 months
may be required in period 2. Furthermore, since the patients starting active
therapy at the end of period 1 are more advanced, the drug may not have
the same effectiveness, nor will the ADAS-Cog necessarily behave in the
same fashion. This will make interpretation of period 2 results difficult. The
sigmoidal nature of the disease-progression curve (as measured by the
ADAS-Cog) will affect in this way, all designs which start active treatment in
period 2 after differential treatment in period 1.

For these reasons, the withdrawal designs (randomized or nonrandom-
ized) may be preferable to delayed starts.

Complete two-period designs

One further design, which is a combination of the randomized withdrawal
design and the randomized delayed-start design, has been discussed for
separating disease-modifying from symptomatic effects in a trial of propentofylline in AD.[73]

This four-arm design is complete in the sense of having an arm for each
sequential combination of active and placebo in two periods (see Figure 7.6).
It allows a more complete understanding of the behavior of a study drug,
avoids unblinding in period 2, and allows estimation of the total period-2

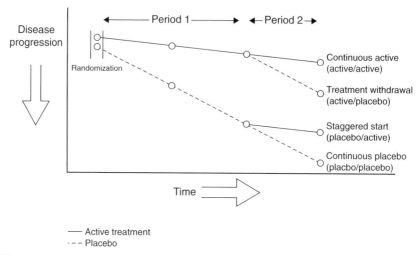

Figure 7.6

Complete two-period design.

treatment effect, and, because patients have a 3:1 chance of being exposed to active drug for at least part of the study, it should result in easier recruitment and better retention of patients than the withdrawal design. In addition, for similar power for inference about the disease-modification and symptomatic treatment effects, the sample size required for such a design is comparable to that of the two-arm withdrawal and staggered-start designs and smaller than that of the randomized-withdrawal and randomized-start designs.

These characteristics, and the significant fact that it also allows much more complete testing of statistical model assumptions needed for trial analysis than the other two-period designs, recommend the complete two-period design for serious consideration for future disease-modification trials in AD.[74]

Mild cognitive impairment—another target of disease-modifying therapies

By the time patients present with AD, the pathologic process is already well established, and neuropsychological dysfunction is clearly evident. To maximally preserve function, intervention earlier in the pathologic process, prior to the development of frank dementia, would be preferable. Furthermore, it is plausible that a window of opportunity exists during which a patient must be treated to be able to respond to a particular disease-modifying agent. The data for anti-inflammatory medications would support this. While multiple epidemiologic studies have indicated that patients who take nonsteroidal anti-inflammatory agents have a lower incidence of AD,[80–83] therapeutic trials of such agents have been disappointing.[84,85]

This might imply that the earlier the intervention in the disease process, the greater the likelihood that it will be effective. If this were true, intervention at a point prior to the establishment of AD would be preferable. Since the rate of development of AD in an asymptomatic elderly population is low (approximately 1% per year),[86] the choice of a mild cognitive impairment (MCI) patient population might offer a viable alternative. Patients with MCI develop dementia at a rate of 10–15% per year,[86] therefore, a demonstration of thera-peutic effect would require a reasonable number of patients (Table 7.3).

In addition, since no effective medication has been approved for symptomatic treatment of MCI, placebo-controlled trials are acceptable to ethics committees, patients, and caregivers alike. A parallel-group design with a placebo washout (as in the withdrawal design above) would be preferable. This design would involve a survival analysis with development of dementia of the Alzheimer type as the primary endpoint.

If the proportion of patients developing AD by the end of period 1 was lower in the active treatment group, either a symptomatic or a disease-modifying effect might be responsible. If the difference is maintained at the end of period 2, which for most compounds would not need to be longer than 3 months, disease modification could be inferred. As with this design in AD, it would be advisable to keep some patients on active therapy during segment 2 to avoid loss of blinding.

If disease modification is demonstrated by this approach, this would allow estimation of very meaningful numbers—delay in development of dementia

Table 7.3. Sample size calculation for MCI trials.

Reduction in conversion to AD	Number per group*	
	24 Months* (12-month accrual, 12-month follow-up)	36 months** (12-month accrual, 24-month follow-up)
Assuming placebo yearly rate of conversion of 12%		
25%	1411	909
33%	671	435
50%	201	133
Assuming placebo yearly rate of conversion of 15%		
25%	1108	727
33%	532	352
50%	161	109

* alpha = 0.05 using a two-sided log rank test with 80% power and two groups
** assuming 40% dropout

and number needed to treat to prevent the development of one case of dementia.

Surrogate endpoints/biological markers in disease-modification trials

Surrogate endpoints may also prove to be powerful tools to support a claim of disease modification. While regulatory acceptance of a surrogate endpoint would not prevent the need for long trials with large numbers of patients, it would permit the use of a more simplified trial design. Even more important-ly, however, it would allow more rapid determination of both proof of concept and dose finding. This would reduce the enormous expenditure of time and money that is otherwise necessary to answer these questions.

An ideal surrogate marker for use in a clinical trial should have several important characteristics. It should be noninvasive, reliable, able to detect a fundamental feature of the neuropathologic process, and sensitive to change over a reasonable time period. In addition, it should correlate with important clinical outcomes in different stages of the pathologic process. While there is no one measure which has received acceptance among either the academic community or regulatory agencies, there are some which show promise.

To date, none of the potential biomarkers that require sampling of cere-brospinal fluid (Aβ42 and tau, and neuronal thread protein) have been adequately studied to determine whether they have sufficient sensitivity, specificity, and correlation with disease severity to prove useful in clinical tri-als. Widespread acceptability of repeated lumbar puncture by patients eligible for a clinical trial is unlikely; therefore, these measures will probably never prove useful as surrogate endpoints in disease-modification studies. Insufficient information is currently available to recommend any plasma or urine biological marker.

Currently, neuroimaging offers the most promise as a surrogate endpoint for disease modification trials for AD. Hippocampal and whole-brain atrophy are all well-known accompaniments of the pathologic process of AD and are related to neuronal loss.[87–89] Since neuronal loss is the final step in the pathologic process, any intervention which delays the progression of AD would presumably affect the progression of atrophy, providing good face validity for these outcomes. Furthermore, since neuronal loss and atrophy are the final result, virtually any disease-modifying agent could use such an outcome measure. This is not necessarily the case for other, nonimaging potential surrogate markers.

Rates of hippocampal atrophy[87,90,91] and rates of various measures of whole-brain atrophy (lateral ventricular volume,[92,93] ventricle-to-brain ratio,[21,94] total cortex,[94] and cerebrospinal fluid volume in ventricular sys-tem[95]) have been reported, and correlation has also been shown between the degree of atrophy and clinical status for some of these measures. Volumetric MRI has been used to demonstrate that cortical atrophy is an index of disease severity in AD and that hippocampal atrophy, in patients without lacunae predicts cognitive decline, further supporting the use of MRI outcomes for this purpose.[96]

Measures of hippocampal volume may offer the most benefit in earlier stages of the pathologic process, particularly in MCI. Hippocampal atrophy predicts MCI patients at higher risk of progression to AD, and requiring hippocampal atrophy at study entry may offer a way to enrich the sample in these trials.[10,96] This would increase the proportion of patients who develop AD and would permit either a shorter trial, a smaller sample size, or the ability to demonstrate a smaller effect size. In addition, rates of hippocampal atrophy have been shown to correlate with clinical status[87] in both MCI and AD, confirming the potential for this outcome to be sensitive to change in these populations. Because hippocampal volume loss occurs relatively early in the clinical course of the pathologic process, it may be that, at later stages, sensitivity of this outcome will be lost. This is speculative, however, since no published literature exists on this topic. Furthermore, since the focus of disease modification is unlikely to include moderately advanced cases, this will not be problematic.

Measures of whole-brain volume also show much promise in this area. Serial MRI over 1 year has been used to look at rates of atrophy in AD patients.[88] A 2.37% (1.11% standard deviation) loss of whole-brain volume over 1 year compared with 0.41% (0.47% standard deviation) in age-matched normal controls was reported. Using these data, the author determined that, correcting for rate of atrophy in normal controls, and assuming a 10% dropout rate and that 10% of scan pairs would be inadequate for analysis, it would take 207 patients per arm to demonstrate a 20% reduction in the rate of atrophy over 1 year with 90% power. A reduction of 30% in the rate of atrophy would require only 92 patients per arm.[88]

In another serial MRI study, a similar rate of whole-brain atrophy over the course of 12 months in mild to moderate AD patients (2.14%, SD 0.52) was reported.[21] This study also examined the change of ventricle-to-brain ratio over this time and found a 15.6% per year rate of decline (SD 2.8%), compared with 4.3% (SD 1.1%) among controls. By this more sensitive measure of brain atrophy, it was estimated that for a 6-month trial, 135 patients per arm would be required to demonstrate a 20% reduction in excess cerebral atrophy or 61 patients per arm to show a 30% reduction.

Irrespective of choice of MRI surrogate endpoint, in a multicenter clinical trial, careful attention to standardizing of MRI capture is critical to success. Methods of both image capture and variable measurement varied widely among reported studies.[21,87,90–94] This must be remembered when designing a study, particularly when determining the sample size. Rates of atrophy and standard deviations cannot be assumed to be similar for different methods of determining these outcomes.

While the available data currently suggest that volumetric MRI may be valuable as a surrogate endpoint in disease-modification trials, there are still a number of unanswered questions which must be addressed.

The literature to date does not report rates of atrophy for all relevant MRI parameters at all stages of the pathologic process (MCI through mild, moderate, and severe dementia). Since these rates may well be stage dependent, this is important information, especially for sample size determinations. In addition, the data that are available need confirmation from further studies, since the patient numbers involved to date have been small. This information is critical for deciding which MRI parameter is best (and at what stage) and also to determine whether absolute volume changes or relative changes are most appropriate. Both the preferred method of image capture and the most reliable method for determining the measurements need to be clarified, as does the minimum time period required for valid results. The sample sizes estimated above assume that the effects on atrophy are immediate. This is probably overly optimistic. Since atrophy represents the final step in the pathologic process, one cannot assume that an intervention which affects an early step in the pathway will have an immediate effect on atrophy.

While these questions remain unanswered, definitive guidance on this issue cannot be given. The information to date, however, would support inclusion of volumetric MRI measurements, on a 6-month basis, in clinical trials of disease modification. Since the largest cost incurred is in the image capture, rather than in the measurement, until the answers are known, measurement of hippocampal and whole-brain volumes, and ventricle-to-brain ratio should be obtained. Rates of atrophy should be calculated both as absolutes and as percentages.

Conclusion

Thus, clinical trials in AD remain in a highly dynamic state. Introduction of novel trial designs, treatment of all patients with cholinesterase inhibitors, close attention to test validations and translation, use of centralized scoring, and inclusion of new, surrogate endpoints will become a standard part of the clinical trials repertoire in the years to come.

References

1. Rogers SL, Farlow MR, Doody RS et al. A 24-week, double-blind, placebo-controlled trial of donepezil in patients with Alzheimer's disease. Neurology 1998; 50:136–145.

2. Burns A, Gauthier S, Perdomo C, Pratt RD. Donepezil provides long-term clinical benefits for patients with Alzheimer's disease. World Alzheimer Congress 1999; 10:237–244.

3. Rogers SL, Doody RS, Pratt RD, Leni JR. Long-term efficacy and safety of donepezil in the treatment of Alzheimer's disease: final analysis of a US multicentre open-label study. Eur Neuropsychopharmacol 2000; 10:195–203.

4. Raskind MA, Peskind ER, Wessel T, Yuan W. Galantamine in AD: a 6-month randomized, placebo-controlled trial with a 6-month extension. The Galantamine USA-1 Study Group. Neurology 2002; 54: 2261–2268.

5. Wilcock GK, Lilienfeld S, Gaens E. Efficacy and safety of galantamine in patients with mild to moderate Alzheimer's disease: multicentre randomised controlled trial. BMJ 2000; 321:1445–1449.

6. Doraiswamy PM, Krishnan KR, Anand R. Long-term effects of rivastigmine in moderately severe Alzheimer's disease: does early initiation of therapy offer sustained benefits? Prog Neuropsychopharmacol Biol Psychiatry 2002; 26:705–712.

7. Kumar V, Anand R, Messina J et al. An efficacy and safety analysis of Exelon in Alzheimer's disease patients with concurrent vascular risk factors. Eur J Neurol 2000; 7:159–169.

8. Knopman DS, Kahn J, Miles S. Clinical research designs for emerging treatments for Alzheimer disease. Arch Neurol 1998; 55:1425–1429.

9. Allain H, Bentue-Ferrer D, Belliard S et al. Mild cognitive impairment: potential therapeutics. Rev Neurol 2002; 158(10 Suppl):S35–S40.

10. Grundman M, Sencakova D, Jack CR et al. Brain MRI hippocampal volume and prediction of clinical status in a mild cognitive impairment trial. J Mol Neurosci 2002; 19:23–27.

11. Feldman H, Gauthier S, Hecker J et al. A 24-week, randomized, double-blind study of donepezil in moderate to severe Alzheimer's disease. Neurology 2001; 57:613–620.

12. McKhann G, Drachman DA, Folstein M et al. Clinical diagnosis of Alzheimer's disease: report of the NINDS–ADRDA Work Group under the auspices of Department of Health and Human Services Task Force on Alzheimer's Disease. Neurology 1984; 34:939–944.

13. Varma AR, Snowden JS, Lloyd JJ et al. Evaluation of the NINCDS–ADRDA criteria in the differentiation of Alzheimer's disease and frontotemporal dementia. J Neurol Neurosurg Psychiatry 1999; 66:184–188.

14. Mann UM, Mohr E, Gearing M, Chase TN. Heterogeneity in Alzheimer's disease: progression rate segregated by distinct neuropsychological and cerebral metabolic profiles. J Neurol Neurosurg Psychiatry 1992; 55:956–959.

15. Marra C, Silveri MC, Gainotti G. Predictors of cognitive decline in the early stage of probable Alzheimer's disease. Dement Geriatr Cogn Disord 2000; 11:212–218.

16. Lopez O, Becker J, Klunk W et al. Research evaluation and diagnosis of probable Alzheimer's disease over the last two decades. I. Neurology 2000; 55:1854–1862.

17. Folstein MF, Folstein SE, McHugh PR. 'Mini-Mental State'. A practical method for grading the cognitive

state of patients for the clinician. J Psychiat Res 1975; 12:189–198.

18. Zec RF, Landreth ES, Vicari SK et al. Alzheimer disease assessment scale: useful for both early detection and staging of dementia of the Alzheimer type. Alzheimer Dis Assoc Disord 1992; 6:89–102.

19. Londos E, Passant U, Gustafson L, Brun A. Neuropathological correlates to clinically defined dementia with Lewy bodies. Int J Geriatr Psychiatry 2001; 16:667–679.

20. Willmer J, Mohr E. Evaluation of selection criteria used in Alzheimer's disease clinical trials. Can J Neurol Sci 1998; 25:39–43.

21. Bradley K, Bydder G, Budge M et al. Serial brain MRI at 3–6 month intervals as a surrogate marker for Alzheimer's disease. Br J Radiol 2002; 75:506–513.

22. Jack C, Slomkowski M, Gracon S et al. MRI as a biomarker of disease progression in a therapeutic trial of milameline for AD. Neurology 2003; 60:253–260.

23. Gibson G, Huang H. Oxidative processes in the brain and non-neuronal tissues as biomarkers of Alzheimer's disease. Front Biosci 2002; 7:d1007-d1015.

24. Khachaturian ZS. The challenges of developing and validating molecular and biochemical markers of Alzheimer's disease. Neurobiol Aging 2002; 23:509–511.

25. Csernansky JG, Miller JP, McKeel D et al. Relationships among cerebrospinal fluid biomarkers in dementia of the Alzheimer type. Alzheimer Dis Assoc Disord 2002; 16:114–149.

26. Diaz-Arrastia R, Baskin F. New biochemical markers in Alzheimer disease. Arch Neurol 2001; 58:354–356.

27. Lopez OL, Becker JT, Klunk W et al. Research evaluation and diagnosis of possible Alzheimer's disease over the last two decades. II. Neurology 2000; 55:1863–1869.

28. Salmon DP, Thomas RG, Pay MM et al. Alzheimer's disease can be accurately diagnosed in very mildly impaired individuals. Neurology 2002; 59:1022–1028.

29. Cummings JL, Khachaturian ZS. Definitions and diagnostic criteria. In: Gauthier S, ed. Clinical Diagnosis and Management of Alzheimers's Disease, 2nd edn. London: Martin Dunitz, 1999: 3–13.

30. Mohr E, Dastoor D, Claus J. Neuropsychological assessment. In: Gauthier S, ed. Clinical Diagnosis and Management of Alzheimers's Disease, 2nd edn. London: Martin Dunitz, 1999: 93–106.

31. Eastley R, Wilcock G. Assessment and differential diagnosis of dementia. In: O'Brien J, Ames D, Burns A, eds. Dementia. Oxford: Oxford University Press, 2000: 41–47.

32. Ashley RV, Gladsjo A, Olson R et al. Changes in psychiatric diagnoses from admission to discharge: review of the charts of 159 patients consecutively admitted to a geriatric psychiatry inpatient unit. Gen Hosp Psychiatry 2001; 23:3–7.

33. Rosen WG, Mohs RC, Davis KL. A new rating scale for Alzheimer's disease. Am J Psychiatry 1984; 141:1356–1364.

34. Imbimbo BP. Pharmacodynamic-tolerability relationships of cholinesterase inhibitors for Alzheimer's disease. CNS Drugs 2001; 15:375–390.

35. Stern RG, Mohs RC, Davidson MH et al. A longitudinal study of Alzheimer's disease: measurement, rate, and predictors of cognitive deterioration. Am J Psychiatry 1994; 151:390–396.

36. Schmeidler J, Mohs RC, Aryan M. Relationship of disease severity to decline on specific cognitive and functional measures in Alzheimer disease. Alzheimer Dis Assoc Disord 1998; 12:146–151.

37. Doraiswamy PM, Kaiser L, Bieber F, Garman RL. The Alzheimer's Disease Assessment Scale: evaluation of psychometric properties and patterns of cognitive decline in multicenter clinical trials of mild to moderate Alzheimer's disease. Alzheimer Dis Assoc Disord 2001; 15:174–183.

38. Corey-Bloom J. The ABC of Alzheimer disease cognitive changes and their management in Alzheimer's disease and related dementias. International Psychogeriatrics 2002; 14 (Suppl 1):51–75.

39. Schmitt FA, Ashford W, Ernesto C et al. The severe impairment battery: concurrent validity and the assessment of longitudinal change in Alzheimer's disease. Alzheimer Dis Assoc Disord 1997; 11(Suppl 2):S51–S56.

40. Schneider LS, Olin JT, Doody RS et al. Validity and reliability of the Alzheimer's Disease Cooperative Study—clinical global impression of change. Alzheimer Dis Assoc Disord 1997; 11(Suppl 2):S22–S32.

41. Schneider LS, Olin JT. Clinical global impressions in Alzheimer's clinical trials. Psychogeriatrics 1996; 8:277–288; discussion 288–290.

42. Hughes CP, Berg L, Danziger WL et al. A new clinical scale for the staging of dementia. Br J Psychiatry 1982; 140:566–572.

43. Burke WJ, Miller JP, Rubin EH et al. Reliability of the Washington University Clinical Dementia Rating. Arch Neurol 1988; 45:31–32.

44. Dooneief G, Marder K, Tang MX, Stern Y. The Clinical Dementia Rating scale: community-based validation of 'profound' and 'terminal' stages. Neurology 1996; 46:1746–1749.

45. Fillenbaum GG, Peterson B, Morris JC. Estimating the validity of the clinical Dementia Rating Scale: the CERAD experience. Consortium to Establish a Registry for Alzheimer's Disease. Aging (Milano) 1996; 8:379–385.

46. Galasko D, Edland SD, Morris JC et al. The Consortium to Establish a Registry for Alzheimer's Disease (CERAD). Part XI. Clinical milestones in patients with Alzheimer's disease followed over 3 years. Neurology 1995; 45:1451–1455.

47. Morris JC. The Clinical Dementia Rating (CDR): current version and scoring rules. Neurology 1993; 43:2412–2414.

48. Morris JC, Ernesto C, Schafer K et al. Clinical dementia rating training and reliability in multicenter studies: the Alzheimer's Disease Cooperative Study experience. Neurology 1997; 48:1508–1510.

49. Morris JC, Heyman A, Mohs RC et al. The Consortium to Establish a Registry for Alzheimer's Disease (CERAD). I. Clinical and neuropsychological assessment of Alzheimer's disease. Neurology 1989; 39:1159–1165.

50. Morris JC, Edland S, Clark C et al. The Consortium to Establish a

Registry for Alzheimer's Disease (CERAD). IV. Rates of cognitive change in the longitudinal assessment of probable Alzheimer's disease. Neurology 1993; 43:2457–2465.

51. Berg L, Miller JP, Baty J et al. Mild senile dementia of the Alzheimer type. IV. Evaluation of intervention. Ann Neurol 1992; 31:242–249.

52. European Agency for the Evaluation of Medicinal Products. CPMP/ EWP/553/95. Note for guidance on medicinal products in the treatment of Alzheimer's disease. Available at www.emea.eu.int/pdfs/human/ewp /055395en.pdf.

53. Gelinas I, Gauthier L, McIntyre M, Gauthier S. Development of a functional measure for persons with Alzheimer's disease: the disability assessment for dementia. Am J Occup Ther 1999; 53:471–481.

54. Feldman H, Santu A, Donald A et al. The disability assessment for dementia scale: a 12-month study of functional ability in mild to moderate severity Alzheimer disease.. Alzheimer Dis Assoc Disord 2001; 15:89–95.

55. Cummings JL, Mega M, Gray K et al. The Neuropsychiatric Inventory: comprehensive assessment of psychopathology in dementia. Neurology 1994; 44:2308–2314.

56. Reisberg B, Borenstein J, Salob SP et al. Behavioral symptoms in Alzheimer's disease: phenomenology and treatment. J Clin Psychiatry 1987; 48 (Suppl):9–15.

57. Deutsch LH, Bylsma FW, Rovner BW et al. Psychosis and physical aggression in probable Alzheimer's disease, Am J Psychiatry 1991; 148:1159–1163.

58. Morriss RK, Rovner BW, Folstein MF, German PS. Delusions in newly admitted residents of nursing homes. Am J Psychiatry 1990; 147:299–302.

59. Steele C, Rovner B, Chase GA, Folstein M. Psychiatric symptoms and nursing home placement of patients with Alzheimer's disease. Am J Psychiatry 1990; 147:1049–1051.

60. Alexopoulos GS, Abrams RC, Young RC, Shamoian CA. Cornell Scale for Depression in Dementia. Biol Psychiatry 1988; 23:271–284.

61. Burke WJ, Houston MJ, Boust SJ, Roccaforte WH. Use of the Geriatric Depression Scale in dementia of the Alzheimer type. J Am Geriatr Soc 1989; 37:856–860.

62. Bohac DL, Smith GE, Rummans TR. Sensitivity, specificity, and predictive value of the Geriatric Depression Scale—Short Form (GDS–SF) among cognitively impaired elderly. Arch Clin Neuropsychol 1996; 11:370 (Abstract).

63. Moore A, McQuay H. Numbers needed to treat derived from meta analysis. NNT is a tool, to be used appropriately. BMJ 1999; 319:1200.

64. Wimo A, Jönsson B, Karlsson G, Winblad B. Health Economics of Dementia. Chichester: Wiley, 1998.

65. Morris JC, Heyman A, Mohs RC et al. The Consortium to Establish a Registry for Alzheimer's Disease (CERAD). I. Clinical and neuropsychological assessment of Alzheimer's disease. Neurology 1989; 39:1159–1165.

66. Peña-Casanova J, Aguilar M, Bertran-Serra I et al. Normalización de instrumentos cognitivos y fun-

cionales para la evaluación de la demencia (NORMACODEM). I. objetivos, contenidos y población. Neurologia 1997; 12:61–68.

67. McDaniel D, Lansink J. Effective investigator meetings. Appl Clin Trials 2001; 10:54–58.

68. Sherretts S, Gard G, Langner H. Frequency of clerical errors on WISC protocols. Psychol Sch 1979; 16:495–496.

69. Freedman B. Equipoise and the ethics of clinical research. N Engl J Med 1987; 317:151–145.

70. Leber P. Slowing the progression of Alzheimer disease: methodologic issues. Alzheimer Dis Assoc Disord 1997; 11(Suppl 5):S10–S21.

71. Bodick N, Forette F, Hadler D et al. Protocols to demonstrate slowing of Alzheimer disease progression. Position paper from the International Working Group on Harmonization of Dementia Drug Guidelines. Alzheimer Dis Assoc Disord 1997; 11(Suppl 3):50–53.

72. Rossor MN, Fox NC, Freeborough PA, Roques PK. Slowing the progression of Alzheimer disease: monitoring progression. Alzheimer Dis Assoc Disord 1997; 11(Suppl 5):S6–9.

73. Whitehouse PJ, Kittner B, Roessner M et al. Clinical trial designs for demonstrating disease-course-altering effects in dementia. Alzheimer Dis Assoc Disord 1998; 12:281–294.

74. McDermott MP, Hall WJ, Oakes D, Eberly S. Design and analysis of two-period studies of potentially disease-modifying treatments. Control Clin Trials 2002; 23:635–649.

75. Tariot PN. Maintaining cognitive function in Alzheimer disease: how effective are current treatments?

Alzheimer Dis Assoc Disord 2001; 15(Suppl 1):S26–S33.

76. Imbimbo BP, Verdelli G, Martelli P, Marchesini D. Two-year treatment of Alzheimer's disease with eptastigmine. The Eptastigmine Study Group. Dement Geriatr Cogn Disord 1999; 10:139–147.

77. Kittner B, Rossner M, Rother M. Clinical trials in dementia with propentofylline. Ann N Y Acad Sci 1997; 826:307–316.

78. Thal LJ, Calvani M, Amato A, Carta A, for the Acetyl-L-Carnitine Study Group. A 1-year controlled trial of acetyl-L-carnitine in early-onset AD. Neurology 2000; 55:805–810.

79. Wimo A, Winblad B, Engedal K et al. An economic evaluation of donepezil in mild to moderate Alzheimer's disease: results of a 1-year, double-blind, randomized trial. Dement Geriatr Cogn Disord 2003; 15:44–54.

80. Rich JB, Rasmusson DX, Folstein MF et al. Nonsteroidal anti-inflammatory drugs in Alzheimer's disease. Neurology 1995; 45:51–55.

81. Breitner JC, Welsh KA, Helms MJ et al. Delayed onset of Alzheimer's disease with nonsteroidal anti-inflammatory and histamine H_2 blocking drugs. Neurobiol Aging 1995; 16:523–530.

82. Andersen K, Launer LJ, Ott A et al. Do nonsteroidal anti-inflammatory drugs decrease the risk for Alzheimer's disease? The Rotterdam Study. Neurology 1995; 45:1441–1445.

83. Stewart WF, Kawas C, Corrada M, Metter EJ. Risk of Alzheimer's disease and duration of NSAID use. Neurology 1997; 48:626–632.

84. Scorer CA. Preclinical and clinical challenges in the development of disease-modifying therapies for Alzheimer's disease. Drug Discov Today 2001; 6:1207–1219.

85. Doraiswamy PM. Non-cholinergic strategies for treating and preventing Alzheimer's disease. CNS Drugs 2002; 16:811–824.

86. Petersen RC, Smith GE, Waring SC et al. Mild cognitive impairment: clinical characterization and outcome. Arch Neurol 1999; 56:303–308.

87. Jack CR, Petersen RC, Xu Y et al. Rates of hippocampal atrophy correlate with change in clinical status in aging and AD. Neurology 2000; 55:484–489.

88. Fox NC, Warrington EK, Rossor MN. Serial magnetic resonance imaging of cerebral atrophy in preclinical Alzheimer's disease. Lancet 1999; 353:2125.

89. Fox NC, Cousens S, Scahill R et al. Using serial registered brain magnetic resonance imaging to measure disease progression in Alzheimer disease: power calculations and estimates of sample size to detect treatment effects. Arch Neurol 2000; 57:339–344.

90. Jack CR Jr, Petersen RC, Xu Y. Hippocampal atrophy and apolipoprotein E genotype are independently associated with Alzheimer's disease. Ann Neurol 1998; 43:303–310.

91. Kaye JA, Swihart T, Howieson D. Volume loss of the hippocampus and temporal lobe in healthy elderly persons destined to develop dementia. Neurology 1997; 48:1297–1304.

92. Luxenberg JS, Haxby JV, Creasey H et al. Rate of ventricular enlargement in dementia of the Alzheimer type correlates with rate of neuropsychological deterioration. Neurology 1987; 37:1135–1140.

93. DeCarli C, Haxby JV, Gillette JA et al. Longitudinal changes in lateral ventricular volume in patients with dementia of the Alzheimer type. Neurology 1992; 42:2029–2036.

94. Burns A, Jacoby R, Levy R. Computed tomography in Alzheimer's disease: a longitudinal study. Biol Psychiatry 1991; 29:383–390.

95. Shear PK, Sullivan EV, Mathalon DH et al. Longitudinal volumetric computed tomographic analysis of regional brain changes in normal aging and Alzheimer's disease. Arch Neurol 1995; 52:392–402.

96. Mungas D, Reed BR, Jagust WJ et al. Volumetric MRI predicts rate of cognitive decline related to AD and cerebrovascular disease. Neurology 2002; 59:867–873.

8
Ethics of research in dementia

Jason Karlawish

The neurodegenerative diseases that cause dementia are common, especially in industrialized nations whose population is aging.[1] They cause substantial morbidity both to the people with dementia and to the people who care for them, typically a family member.[2,3] Extensive research efforts are underway to address these problems. The success of these research efforts rests in large part on the effective enrollment of persons with dementia as research subjects.

There are two key ethical requirements for the responsible conduct of research: informed consent from the subject,[4(45CFR46.116)] and the judgment that the risks of research are reasonable with respect to the potential benefits, if any, to subjects and to the expectation that the research will yield important knowledge.[4(45CFR46.111(a)(2))] But the very problems caused by dementia that warrant research are also the cause of ethical challenges to investigators and institutional review boards (IRBs) to fulfill these requirements. The patients' early and progressive cognitive impairments significantly hinder their ability to give informed consent and complicate the problem of consensus on the kinds of risks that are reasonable in the pursuit of important knowledge.[5–8]

The core challenge in research that involves persons with dementia is defining acceptable conditions under which to expose a noncompetent person to the risks, burdens, or discomforts of an intervention that is intended not to benefit that person but to produce generalizable knowledge that will benefit other people. For the past 30 years, national governments and investigators have struggled to articulate a coherent set of principles and rules.[9] The struggle has been how to integrate the principles of respect for autonomy, beneficence, and justice into a coherent set of safeguards that allows valuable research to proceed without offending the subjects' rights and dignity. This lengthy effort has produced a set of core safeguards: decision-making capacity assessment, respect for patient assent and dissent, proxy decision-making, risk–benefit assessment, and evidence of the subjects' preferences.[10] This chapter reviews the justification for each of these safeguards and describes techniques that investigators and IRBs can use to implement them.

Decision-making capacity assessment

A key ethical principle that ensures the responsible conduct of clinical research is respect for subject autonomy.[11–13] It demands of an investigator two responsibilities: to ensure that a subject's decision reflects his or her goals and values, and to protect a subject who cannot make a decision from making it. The means to fulfill these responsibilities is informed consent.[4,14(§46.116)]

Informed consent is a process with two steps: disclosure and assessment of decision-making capacity. During disclosure, the investigator reviews the informed-consent form with the potential subject. This review is essentially a teaching session in which the investigator reviews eight core elements, as summarized in Table 8.1. Next, the investigator assesses the subject's decision-making capacity in order to decide whether the subject is competent to make the decision of whether to enroll in the research.

The terms 'decision-making capacity' and 'competency' have been used with various and even interchangeable meanings. Decision-making capacity, or 'capacity,' consists of the abilities to understand, appreciate, reason, and choose. Their definitions are as follows:[15] understanding is the ability to comprehend the meaning of information disclosed; appreciation is the ability to recognize how information applies to one's own personal situation; reasoning is the ability to compare options (comparative reasoning) and to infer consequences of choices (consequential reasoning); and choice is the ability to state consistently a decision.

A key distinction is that between the concepts of understanding and appreciation. Understanding describes the ability to know what information means. In contrast, appreciation describes the ability to apply that information to one's own situation. Whereas understanding assesses a person's ability to know facts, appreciation assesses people's ability to integrate those facts into their goals, values, and beliefs. Hence, a person can understand that drug assignment is randomized but fail to appreciate that the study physician will not get to choose what drug he or she receives ('They give it out by flipping a coin, but Dr Jones will see to it I get what I need'). Deficits in appreciation can be the result of patently false beliefs, delusions, or psychotic states.

Decision-making capacity can be measured in the same way that a skilled clinician can measure a patient's mood or short-term memory. An instrument such as the MacArthur Competency Assessment Tool for Clinical Research (MacCAT-CR) allows the investigator to fit the details of a protocol into open-ended questions that assess these abilities.[6,8,16] Table 8.1 shows a set of standard questions that an investigator can use to assess a subject's decision-making abilities.

The value of a decision-making capacity assessment is that it informs a judgment of competency. Competency describes a judgment about a person's capacity. Specifically, it means a person has adequate decision-making

Table 8.1. A summary of the steps of informed consent and how to achieve them.

Disclosure	Assessment of capacity
The investigator sits side by side with the subject and reviews the informed-consent form.	The investigator asks the subject questions that assess the subject's abilities to make a decision.

Elements that should be disclosed. Note that this list of elements can be altered. US regulations detail conditions for altering this (46.116(c–d)).

(1) A statement that the study involves research; an explanation of the purpose, duration, procedures with attention to any procedures that are experimental or not part of the standard of care

(2) Description of reasonably foreseeable risks or discomforts

(3) Description of benefits to the subject or to others that can reasonably be expected

(4) Description of appropriate alternatives to enrolling

(5) Statement of how confidentiality will be maintained

(6) Explanation of compensation and treatment for research-related injuries

(7) Whom to contact for questions and in the event of an injury

(8) A statement that enrollment in voluntary

Decision-making abilities, definitions, and model questions to assess them. Adapted from the MacArthur Competency Assessment Tool for Clinical Research.[16]

Understanding: the ability to comprehend the meaning of information disclosed.

'Can you tell me in your own words what [are/is] the [summarize the item disclosed]?', eg the benefits of this research or the purpose of this research.

Appreciation: the ability to recognize how information applies to one's own situation.

Appreciate benefit to society: 'Do you believe you have been asked to enroll in this research for your own personal benefit?'

Appreciate risk: 'Do you think it is possible that this research could cause you harm?'

Appreciate randomization: 'Will any of your own personal medical needs determine whether you get the drug or the placebo?'

Similar questions can be formulated to assess appreciation of other relevant items as dictated by the protocol.

Reasoning: the ability logically to manipulate information.

Comparative reasoning: 'How is enrolling in this research better than not enrolling in it?'

Consequential reasoning: 'How might being in this research affect your personal and everyday activities?'

Choice: the ability to state a decision consistently.

'Do you think you are more likely to want to enroll or not to enroll in this research?

capacity to make a decision.[17–19] Competency is often considered a legal judgment, but, in practice, assessments of decision-making capacity are used to make de facto judgments of patient competency to make a particular decision. such as enrolling in research.[17,19,20] Competency is a categorical condition. A person either is or is not competent.

Research on competency shows mixed results in interrater agreement in judgments of competency.[21–23] However, when raters are provided with guidance on the measures of capacity, and they review a structured capacity interview, there is generally good interrater agreement.[6,24] Sources of disagreement will include differences in the weight the competency judge applies to errors that a person makes. For example, a judge may consider the failure to understand the randomization to placebo a critical error. In contrast, another judge may simply require that the subject know that there is a chance of a placebo, but the subject need not understand the procedure by which he or she might get it. Recognizing these differences among judges, an investigator team may decide in advance the core performance a subject needs to have on measures of decision-making capacity in order to be competent.

Studies of the capacity and competency of persons with dementia have largely focused on Alzheimer's disease (AD). Among patients with mild to early moderate AD (Mini-Mental State Examination [MMSE] scores of ≥18),[25] the reported ranges of the proportion who have at least marginal capacity to understand are 5–73%; to appreciate, 32–100%; and to reason, 50–82%.[5,6,8] These ranges in performance by persons with dementia illustrate that dementia clearly affects a person's ability to make a decision. The primary causes of impairments in AD patient performance are deficits in executive function and language.[26] The informed-consent form's length and complex language probably worsen these impairments in performance.[27–30]

But there is variation in performance—for example, from 5% to 73%—showing marginal capacity to understand. This variation in ranges probably reflects different methods of administering the assessment. For example, a technique that does not allow subjects to retain written information before them will probably show poor performance on measures of understanding.[5,6] The severity of impairments in short-term memory probably explain this. The subject simply cannot hold on to the information. In contrast, a technique that allows the subjects to retain the information before them will show better performance on understanding.[8]

No studies have examined whether an intervention can benefit persons with AD in the informed-consent process. However, a plausible and testable approach would be as follows. In addition to the informed-consent form, the process should provide subjects with the information in simple, easy-to-understand summary format, such as a one-page sheet that the person can use during the capacity assessment. Such a memory and organizational aid might mitigate the functional consequences of executive dysfunction. Such an aid functions as a cognitive prosthetic because it will help these patients stay focused on the consent session, and find it less confusing and thus not frustrating.

The assessment of understanding should require the subject to comprehend the meaning of the information. Hence, if the summary sheet says, 'The risks of the research are stomach upset and liver injury', the question that assesses understanding of the research risks should ask, 'What are the ways a person in this study might be harmed?'. The substitution of 'harm' for 'risk' and 'study' for 'research' requires the subject to abstract the meaning of the information and not simply parrot what is on the memory and organizational aid. The investigator would then use the results of the assessment of decision-making capacity to make a compendious judgment of the subject's competency to enroll in the research.

Respect for patient assent and dissent

A capacity assessment may show that a person is not competent to make the decision to enroll in the research. Consensus generally exists that the investigator should seek the subject's assent and respect his or her dissent.[9,31–34] But clear consensus does not exist on a standard to assess the ability to assent or to dissent, and no studies report the validity or reliability of standards to assess this ability.

A side-by-side comparison of recommendations and regulations shows great variability in what assent means. The US regulations for research that involve children define 'assent' as 'a child's affirmative agreement to participate in research. Mere failure to object should not, absent affirmative agreement, be construed as assent.'[4(§46.402(b))] This suggests that assent is the ability to choose, which is the simplest of the decision-making abilities. In contrast, proposed US regulations for adults who lack the ability to consent define 'assent' as 'the ability to know (1) what procedures will be performed in the research and that he or she may withdraw from participation, (2) choose freely to undergo these procedures, and (3) communicate this choice unambiguously.'[31(pg.11332)] This standard adds some aspects of the ability to understand to the pediatric requirement of the ability to choose. The Canadian Tri-Council standard is that the subject should 'understand the nature and consequences of the research'.[35(article 2.7)] The point of this side-by-side comparison is that merely saying 'yes' (or 'no') may be insufficient evidence of the ability to assent (or dissent). Some other abilities may be necessary, such as understanding key facts or appreciating key risks. Operationalizing a subject's dissent is ambiguous as well. For example, in dementia research that focuses on agitation and related behavioral disorders, an eligible subject may resist care and say 'no' to any intervention, research, or treatment. Respecting this dissent is illogical.

Because widely accepted standards for assent and dissent are not available, research protocols should describe what kinds of decision-making abilities a person needs to demonstrate to show that he or she can assent or dissent. The informed-consent form should include a section to document these assessments—for example, a checklist to indicate whether the subject adequately understood key items needed to assent. An agitation trial might require that dissent means that the person knows the project is research. Thus, simply saying 'no' is insufficient.

Proxy consent

When subjects are judged not competent, someone else must decide for them. The increasingly vexing issue in proxy consent is the legal authority of a person to serve in this role.[36] This recapitulates a controversy that began in the late 1970s over the authority to withdraw life-sustaining therapy.

US research regulations state that a proxy is a 'legally authorized representative'.[4(45CFR46.116)] However, in the USA, most state laws lack clear guidance on who is legally authorized. California has recently passed a law that designates who can serve as a research proxy.[37] It largely follows the legal approach to proxy decision-making in clinical care. Those laws instruct a clinician to obtain informed consent from a hierarchy of family relationships widely thought to represent 'closeness', such as spouse followed by adult children.[38]

In many instances, this hierarchy also describes the person who is an ethically appropriate surrogate. But, in some cases, the two conditions do not coexist in the same person. An adult grandchild who has lived with, cared for, and made medical decisions for a demented grandparent is arguably in a more ethically appropriate role than the grandparent's estranged child. A family member in such a caregiver role appreciates that research risks and benefits are interdependent between themselves and the subject.[39] Hence, the family member makes a decision that reflects an appreciation of how research risks can affect the patient.

The well-established role of a family caregiver in dementia care means that dementia researchers have a clear person to turn to as a proxy. A protocol should define who is a caregiver. This would include serving as knowledgeable informant for health-care professionals, assisting the person in activities of daily living, and making decisions for or with the person with dementia. When this person is not also the legally authorized representative, the investigator will need to obtain informed consent from both people.

A proposed guideline for proxy consent is that the proxy exercise a substituted judgment, choosing what the patient would choose if they were capable of choosing for themselves.[9] This guideline reflects a strong adherence to the principle of respect for autonomy. It raises concern about the legitimacy of proxy informed consent because a proxy may enroll a subject even though the proxy believes that the subject himself would not want to enroll.[40] But this evidence may not be as morally distressing as it appears. Just as in clinical care, proxies cannot consistently make accurate substituted judgments for research enrollment.[41] The claim 'he would want to enroll' is as likely to be wrong as to be right. In addition, as in clinical care decisions,[42] many potential subjects would grant their proxy leeway over their advance directive to enroll in potentially beneficial research.[43]

Instead of requiring a substituted judgment, a reasonable guideline would require the informed-consent form to instruct the proxy to use the potential subject's previous wishes, and if this information is not available—which is likely the case in most situations—to decide what is in the subject's best interests. This language could appear in a section titled 'instructions for persons acting as a proxy for noncompetent subjects'.

Risk–benefit assessment

The research safeguards above focus on the subject protection of informed consent. It is a core protection in the case of research that involves a competent adult. A competent adult is allowed extensive personal discretion in the decision to enroll in research.[44] But the proxy of a noncompetent adult should not have this same discretion.[9,31–34] The core ethical challenge in dementia research is defining the limits on the kinds of research risks the proxy can permit a noncompetent subject to take. These limits serve two roles. First, they guide the degree of subject protection needed. The greater the risk, the more protection needed. Second, limits on research risk define when it is appropriate to enroll noncompetent subjects.

Pediatric research regulations developed in the USA in the 1970s provide a model for these limits.[4(45CRF46subpartD)] A proxy should be allowed to enroll a person if the IRB finds that the research is potentially beneficial or presents minimal risks and the knowledge that may result will be important to the class of subjects.[9,31–34] These categories formalize the widely held requirement that research risks should be reasonable with respect to the potential benefits to the subjects and the importance of the results the research may yield.[4(45CFR46.111(a)(2))] IRBs and investigators need to make a risk–benefit analysis and a risk–knowledge analysis.

But IRBs and investigators have ambiguous guidance on how to fit research risks and benefits into these categories and how to balance the risks and potential benefits to the subjects, and the risks and the value of the knowledge the research may produce.[45,46] The following case illustrates this ambiguity. The typical dementia clinical trial tests a promising drug on a control group. The new drug may have risks such as liver injury, nausea, vomiting, and brain inflammation. These risks are certainly greater than minimal. How can proxy consent be permissible? However, the drug has promising preclinical data suggesting that it presents potential benefits to the subjects. Which risks are justified by these benefits?

A commonly applied approach compares all of the research risks with all of the potential benefits to the subjects. The judgment that the risks are reasonable with respect to the potential benefits—such as a delay in functional loss—justifies these risks, even though they appear 'greater than minimal'. This approach is intuitively appealing because it reflects clinical reasoning. But it fails to recognize that research typically includes procedures that are not designed to provide subjects with potential benefits. These are procedures done to ensure that the research will produce generalizable knowledge that answers a research question. The risks of these procedures ought to be the focus of the minimal risk assessment for proxy consent.

Suppose the drug trial included a lumbar puncture at the start, middle and end of the research. The purpose of the procedure is to assess how the new drug penetrates into the central nervous system. These data are gathered and analysed in such a way that the treating clinician could not use them to affect patient care. Under these conditions, the spinal tap does not yield data that will potentially improve the subject's care. But the research-risk assessment described above would balance the risks of the lumbar puncture against the potential benefits of the drug. A risk that is part of an intervention done solely to generate generalizable knowledge (the lumbar puncture) is justified by the potential benefits of another research intervention (the drug). This bundling of risks and benefits can exploit vulnerable subjects in the pursuit of knowledge.

A research–risk assessment that avoids these problems distinguishes between risks that are justified by potential benefits to the subjects, and risks that are not justified by those benefits.[45] This framework recognizes that research has two distinct components.[46] One component is interventions that present subjects with both risks and potential benefits (the new drug). The other component is interventions that pose risks but offer no potential benefits to the subjects (the lumbar puncture). A coherent justification of a study's risks separately analyses the risks of these components. The risks of components with potential benefits can be justified only by those components' potential benefits. The risks of components that do not have potential benefits are justified by the importance or value of the knowledge that may reasonably result from the research.[47,48]

How much can that risk be? A useful guidance principle is the concept of minimal risk: 'The probability and magnitude of harm or discomfort anticipated in the research are not greater in and of themselves than those ordinarily encountered in daily life or during the performance of routine physical or psychological examinations or tests.'[4(45CFR46.102(i))] There has been considerable confusion about how to apply this definition because this definition lacks a comparison group whose risks of daily life might be used to compare with the research risks.[49] Options include comparing the research risks with the risks faced in the daily lives of the subjects of the research, the general public, or healthy persons.[45]

Risk assessment is highly contextual. IRBs and investigators should recognize that the group they select changes the degree of risk that they judge 'minimal'. The 'subjects of the research' describes persons with illness who may face significant risks because of their illness. In contrast, 'healthy persons' describes a group whose risks are considerably less than persons who are ill. The general public lies somewhere between. The choice of comparison group should reflect the principle of justice. Vulnerable subjects are not to be exposed to excessive research risks, without the possibility of benefit, in the pursuit of scientific progress.[11]

The two-component model of research–risk assessment described above can help investigators and IRBs judge whether research risks are reasonable with respect to two things: potential benefits, if any, to the subjects, and the importance of the results the research may yield.[4(45CFR46.111(a)(2))] Proxy consent is permissible if the risks of components of the research that do not present potential benefits to the subjects are no more than minimal and are justified by the importance of the knowledge to be gained.

In general, most dementia research will pass the two-component model of research–risk assessment. Components without potential benefits, such as a MRI done to confirm eligibility criteria, present risks no greater than those encountered in routine medical care and tests. In other words, these risks are minimal. They are justified by the importance of the knowledge anticipated from the research. The risks of components with potential benefits, such as the promising new drug, are justified by the state of equipoise: the expert consensus that the interventions being compared are within the standard of care, and that equilibrium exists in the balance of the risks and benefits of the intervention and control groups.[46,50]

In addition to guiding when it is appropriate to obtain proxy consent for research, the two-component model can ensure that the enrollment of demented individuals is necessary. Past research scandals have included recruiting demented persons simply because they were a convenient and available subject population. The two-component model makes plain that research risks that are part of components without potential benefits to the subjects cannot be bundled into a protocol that has potentially beneficial components. Instead, the researchers must justify each component on its own merits.

One class of research that does present an ethical challenge is early-phase research that is designed to assess the safety and toxicity of a drug. This is often greater than minimal risk research, as in double-blind, placebo-controlled, dose-escalation studies done in an inpatient, acute-care facility to assess a new drug's safety and maximum tolerated dose.[51] The risks of these kinds of studies call into question whether the common practice in AD research of caregiver consent and patient assent adequately protects subjects' rights and interests.[32,34,52,53]

What are reasonable resolutions of this issue? One approach would restrict this research to competent subjects. Given that the sample size for these studies is generally small, and that data suggest that about 50% of patients with mild to early moderate AD are competent to consent,[6,8] this proposal may be feasible and properly balance respect for subjects' rights and the societal benefit. A weaker subject protection would require subject assent that fulfills well-defined criteria. For example, the subject will need to state clearly that the research does not offer a direct benefit to his or her health.

Evidence of patients' preferences and interests

Patients with mild to moderate AD are involved in decisions about their medical care and research.[39,54] Hence, the patient may not be able to make the decision, but he or she is voicing preferences and views. These can be valuable data for present as well as future research decisions. Several guidelines have argued that persons with dementia should put these preferences into a research advance directive (RAD). This is modeled on an advance directive for clinical care that instructs a proxy on the kinds of care a person would not want to receive under certain clinical circumstances, such as permanent coma or persistent vegetative state. RADs have been proposed as necessary to enroll a patient in greater than minimal risk research.[9,31–34]

As useful as the concept of a RAD seems, people's attitudes about the uses and value of a RAD suggest a series of paradoxes. A survey of persons with a family history of AD found the vast majority willing to execute a RAD, but when offered the opportunity to execute one, few did so.[43] The majority preferred to have RAD instructions followed over a family member's choice, but the majority also permitted a family member to overrule a RAD in the case of potentially beneficial research.

These results suggest that the following issues need further investigation. First, how would subjects who make RADs want them followed? In particular, how would subjects regard a proxy overriding a RAD instruction not to enroll them in research that is not potentially beneficial? In clinical care, many persons want their best interests taken into consideration with their directive, even if that means overriding the directive.[42] But 'best interests' are an unusual standard in research settings where there is either no plausible individual benefit or no real chance of risk to the research participant. In these situations, 'best interests' might be understandable only as an appreciation of the altruistic intents of either the subject or the proxy. The answers to these issues will not decide whether we should have RADs, but they will go a long way to address the core challenge that raised the need for them in the first place. When is it appropriate to expose a noncompetent person to the risks, burdens, or discomforts of an intervention that is not intended to benefit that person but to produce generalizable knowledge that will benefit other people?

Summary

Research is an essential foundation for the development of rational therapeutics. It is increasingly recognized as a valuable tool for deciding the best way to allocate resources. Inherent in all research is the use of procedures that expose subjects to risks, discomforts, or simply threats to privacy and confidentiality that are not justified by potential benefits to the subjects. In general, society has justified these costs with two kinds of justifications: the subject's personal choice (informed consent) and an institutional research review (IRB review). In the case of research that involves persons who have dementia, informed consent is difficult to obtain, and the clear societal consensus on appropriate research risks is elusive. The protections outlined describe a matrix of subject protections that investigators and IRBs can use to determine what research risks are appropriate and what is an ethical way to enroll subjects who are themselves not capable of consenting to those risks.

References

1. Brookmeyer R, Gray S, Kawas C. Projections of Alzheimer's disease in the United States and the impact of delaying disease onset. Am J Pub Health 1998; 88:1337–1342.

2. Schulz R, O'Brien A, Bookwala J, Fleissner K. Psychiatric and physical morbidity effects of dementia caregiving: prevalence, correlates, and causes. Gerontologist 1995; 35:771–791.

3. Wolfson C, Wolfson DB, Asgharian M et al. A reevaluation of the duration of survival after the onset of dementia. N Engl J Med 2001; 344:1111–1116.

4. Department of Health and Human Services. Common Rule, 45 CFR 46. Federal policy for the protection of human subjects; notices and rules. Fed Reg 1991; 56:28003–28032.

5. Marson DC, Ingram KK, Cody HA, Harrell LE. Assessing the competency of patients with Alzheimer's disease under different legal standards: a prototype instrument. Arch Neurol 1995; 52:949–954.

6. Kim SYH, Caine ED, Currier GW et al. Assessing the competence of persons with Alzheimer's disease in providing informed consent for participation in research. Am J Psychiatry 2001; 158:710–717.

7. Sachs GA, Stocking CB, Stern R et al. Ethical aspects of dementia research: informed consent and proxy consent. Clin Res 1994; 42:403–412.

8. Karlawish JHT, Casarett DJ, James BD. Alzheimer's disease patients' and caregivers' capacity, competency and reasons to enroll in an early phase Alzheimer's disease clinical trial. J Am Geriatr Soc 2002; 50:2019–2024.

9. National Bioethics Advisory Commission. Research Involving Persons with Mental Disorders That May Affect Their Decision-Making Capacity. Vol I. Report and Recommendations. Rockville, MD: US Government Printing Office, 1998: 88.

10. Wendler D, Prasad K. Core safeguards for clinical research with adults who are unable to consent. Ann Intern Med 2001; 135:514–523.

11. National Commission for the Protection of Human Subjects of

Biomedical and Behavioral Research. The Belmont Report: ethical principles and guidelines for the protection of human subjects of research. Fed Reg 1979; 44:23192–23197.

12. Trials of War Criminals Before the Nuremberg Military Tribunals Under Control Council Law No. 10. Vol. 2. Washington, DC: US Government Printing Office, 1949:181–182.

13. World Medical Association. Declaration of Helsinki. Ethical principles for medical research involving human subjects. www.wma.net/policy. World Medical Association, 2000.

14. Faden RR, Beauchamp TL. A History and Theory of Informed Consent. New York: Oxford University Press, 1986:274–297.

15. Grisso T, Appelbaum PS. Assessing Competence to Consent to Treatment. A Guide for Physicians and Other Health Professionals. New York: Oxford University Press, 1998:31–60.

16. Appelbaum PS, Grisso T. The MacArthur Competence Assessment Tool—Clinical Research. Sarasota, FL: Professional Resources Press, 2000.

17. Lo B. Assessing decision-making capacity. Law Med Health Care 1990; 18:193–201.

18. White BC. Competence to Consent. Washington, DC: Georgetown University Press, 1994:44–81.

19. Grisso T, Appelbaum PS. Assessing Competence to Consent to Treatment. A Guide for Physicians and Other Health Professions. New York: Oxford University Press, 1998:127–148.

20. Karlawish JHT, Schmitt FA. Why physicians need to become more proficient in assessing their patients' competency and how they can achieve this [editorial]. J Am Geriatr Soc 2000; 48:1014–1016.

21. Schmand B, Gouwenberg B, Smit JH, Jonker C. Assessment of mental competency in community-dwelling elderly. Alzheimer Dis Assoc Disord 1999; 13:80–87.

22. Fazel S, Hope T, Jacoby R. Assessment of competence to complete advance directives: validation of a patient centered approach. BMJ 1999; 318:493–497.

23. Marson DC, McInturff B, Hawkins L et al. Consistency of physician judgments of capacity to consent in mild Alzheimer's disease. J Am Geriatr Soc 1997; 45:453–457.

24. Marson DC, Earnst KS, Jamil F et al. Consistency of physicians' legal standard and personal judgments of competency in patients with Alzheimer's disease. J Am Geriatr Soc 2000; 48:911–918.

25. Folstein M, Folstein S, McHugh P. Mini-mental state: a practical method for grading the cognitive state of patients for the clinician. J Psychiatr Res 1975; 12:189–198.

26. Marson D, Harrell L. Executive dysfunction and loss of capacity to consent to medical treatment in patients with Alzheimer's disease. Semin Clin Neuropsychol 1999; 4:41–49.

27. Paasche-Orlow MK, Taylor HA, Brancati FL. Readability standards for informed-consent forms as compared with actual readability. N Engl J Med 2003; 348:721–726.

28. White LJ, Jones JS, Felton CW, Pool LC. Informed consent for

medical research: common discrepancies and readability. Acad
Emerg Med 1996; 3:745–750.

29. Morrow GR. How readable are subject consent forms? JAMA 1980;
244:56–58.

30. Grossman SA, Piantadosi S,
Covahey C. Are informed consent
forms that describe clinical oncolo-
gy research protocols readable by
most patients and their families? J
Clin Oncol 1994; 12:2211–2215.

31. Department of Health Education
and Welfare. Protection of human
subjects. Proposed regulations on
research involving those institutionalized as mentally disabled. Fed
Reg 1978; 43:53950–53956.

32. American College of Physicians.
Cognitively impaired subjects [posi-
tion paper]. Ann Intern Med 1989;
111:843–848.

33. Melnick VL, Dubler N, Weisbard A,
Butler RN. Alzheimer's Dementia:
Dilemmas in Clinical Research.
Clifton, NJ: Humana Press,
1985:295–310.

34. Fletcher JC, Dommel W Jr, Cowell
DD. Consent to Research with
Impaired Human Subjects. IRB: A
Review of Human Subjects
Research 1985; 7:1–6.

35. Tri-Council Working Group. Code of
conduct for research involving
humans. (Accessed: 11 July 2002,
at www.ethics.ubc.ca/code/).

36. Hoffman DE, Schwartz J. Proxy
consent to participation of the deci-
sionally impaired in medical
research—Maryland's policy initiative. J Health Care Policy 1998;
1:123–153.

37. State of California. An Act to
Amend Section 24178 of the Health

and Safety Code, Relating to
Health, 2002.

38. American Bar Association.
Surrogate Consent in the Absence
of an Advance Directive, 2001.

39. Karlawish JHT, Casarett D,
Klocinksi J, Sankar P. How do AD
patients and their caregivers decide
whether to enroll in a clinical trial?
Neurology 2001; 56:789–792.

40. Warren JW, Sobal J, Tenney JH et al.
Informed consent by proxy: an issue
in research with elderly patients. N
Engl J Med 1986; 315:1124–1128.

41. Coppolino M, Ackerson L. Do surrogate decision makers provide
accurate consent for intensive care
research? Chest 2001; 119:603–12.

42. Sehgal A, Galbraith A, Chesney M et
al. How strictly do dialysis patients
want their advance directive followed? JAMA 1992; 267:59–63.

43. Wendler D, Martinez RA, Fairclough
D et al. Views of potential subjects
toward proposed regulations for
clinical research with adults unable
to consent. Am J Psychiatry 2002;
159:585–591.

44. Daugherty C, Ratain MJ,
Grochowski E et al. Perceptions of
cancer patients and their physicians
involved in phase 1 trials. J Clin
Oncol 1995; 13:1062–1072.

45. National Bioethics Advisory
Commission. Ethical and Policy
Issues in Research Involving Human
Participants. Vol. I. Report and
Recommendations of the National
Bioethics Advisory Commission.
Bethesda, MD: US Government
Printing Office, 2001:69–96.

46. Weijer C. The ethical analysis of
risk. J Law Med Ethics 2000;
28:344–61.

47. Freedman B. Scientific value and validity as ethical requirements for research: a proposed explication. IRB: A Review of Human Subjects Research 1987; 9:7–10.

48. Casarett D, Karlawish JHT, Moreno JD. A taxonomy of value in clinical research. IRB: Ethics and Human Research 2002; 24:1–6.

49. Karlawish JHT, Hall JB. The controversy over emergency research: a review of the issues and suggestions for a resolution. Am J Respir Crit Care Med 1996; 153:499–506.

50. Freedman B. Equipoise and the ethics of clinical research. N Engl J Med 1987; 317:141–145.

51. Cutler NR, Sramek JJ. Guidelines for conducting bridging studies in Alzheimer disease. Alzheimer Dis Assoc Disord 1998; 12:88–92.

52. Karlawish J, Sachs GA. Research on the cognitively impaired: lessons and warnings from the emergency research debate. J Am Geriatr Soc 1997; 45:474–481.

53. Dresser R. Mentally disabled research subjects: the enduring policy issues. JAMA 1996; 276:67–72.

54. Karlawish JH, Casarett D, Propert KJ et al. Relationship between Alzheimer's disease severity and patient participation in decisions about their medical care. J Geriatr Psychiatry Neurol 2002; 15:68–72.

9
Memantine: A glutamate antagonist for treatment of Alzheimer's disease

Rachelle Smith Doody, Bengt Winblad and
Vesna Jelic

Introduction

There is circumstantial evidence for increased excitotoxicity due to increased glutamatergic stimulation of NMDA receptors in Alzheimer's disease (AD). Pathologic stimulation of glutamatergic receptors results in abnormally high levels of intracellular calcium and, in vitro, may ultimately lead to cell death. The moderate- to low-affinity N-methyl-D-aspartate (NMDA) receptor antagonist, memantine, has shown benefits on cognitive and functional measures compared with placebo in trials of mixed dementia populations and severe AD.[1,2] Memantine has also shown benefit for patients with vascular dementia in double-blind, placebo-controlled studies.[3,4] In the study of a severe, mixed population, memantine was associated with reduced care dependence,[1] and, in the study of patients with severe AD, it was also associated with pharmacoeconomic benefits.[5] The drug was well tolerated, with few or no drug-induced side effects at the doses studied. Although there is no evidence that memantine arrests the progression of AD or mixed AD and vascular dementia (VaD), it appears to slow the progression of disease on multiple outcome measures.

Alzheimer's disease study results

The Benefit and Efficacy in Severely Demented Patients During Treatment with Memantine (M-BEST) study

This study examined the benefits of memantine in institutionalized patients living in seven nursing homes in Riga, Latvia. The study included 166 patients diagnosed with severe dementia whose Mini-Mental State Examination (MMSE)[6] score was less than 10.[1] The baseline characteristics of patients are summarized in Table 9.1.

The trial was designed as a two-arm, double-blind, parallel-group comparison, and randomized patients received either memantine (5 mg/day

Table 9.1. M-BEST patient characteristics at baseline (ITT sample, $n = 166$).

Characteristic	Memantine	Placebo	Total
Sex			
male:female (%)	33:49 (40.2/59.8)	37:47 (44.0/56.0)	70:96 (42.2/57.8)
Age (years) (mean ± SD)			
male	67.7 ± 5.1	69.1 ± 5.8	68.4 ± 5.5
female	73.6 ± 5.8	74.2 ± 5.3	73.9 ± 5.6
BMI (kg/sq m) (mean ± SD)			
male	25.1 ± 3.9	25.8 ± 3.0	25.5 ± 3.5
female	25.9 ± 4.7	25.2 ± 3.7	25.6 ± 4.3
Smokers (%)	22.0	15.5	18.7
Patients (%) with antidementia premedication	39.0	39.3	39.2
Patients (%) with concomitant diseases	87.8	90.5	89.2
Patients (%) with concomitant medication	41.5	42.9	42.2
GDS (cognitive decline) (%)			
moderately severe	3.7	3.6	3.6
severe	91.5	89.3	90.4
very severe	4.9	7.1	6.0
MMSE total score (mean ± SD)	6.6 ± 2.7	6.1 ± 2.8	6.3 ± 2.7
HIS sum score (mean + SD)	5.2 ± 2.9	5.7 ± 3.2	5.5 ± 3.1
HAM-D total score (mean ± SD)	8.5 ± 2.0	8.9 ± 2.1	8.7 ± 2.1
CGI-S (%)			
markedly ill	63	47	55
severely ill	32	39	36
extremely ill	5	13	9
BGP subscore 'care dependence' (mean ± SD)	21.3 ± 7.6	21.8 ± 7.7	21.5 ± 7.6
BGP scores (mean ± SD):			
Agressiveness	2.01 ± 2.2	2.13 ± 2.1	2.07 ± 2.1
Physical disability	2.78 ± 1.8	3.27 ± 2.0	3.03 ± 1.9
Depressive behaviour	2.49 ±1.4	2.81 ± 1.3	2.65 ± 1.4
Neuropsych. disability	3.63 + 1.0	3.51 ± 2.0	3.57 ± 1.9
Inactivity	10.93 ± 2.3	11.42 ± 2.0	11.17 ± 2.1

ITT = intention to treat; SD = standard deviation.

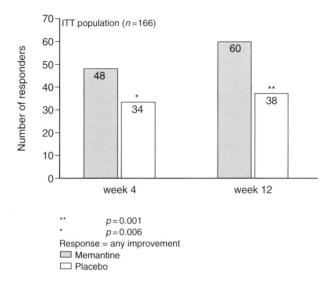

Figure 9.1
M-BEST results in CGI-C.

during the first week and 10 mg/day during the following 11 weeks) or place-bo. The study used measures such as global clinical improvement and validated functional behavioral scales to comply with European CPMP requests for relevant and credible benefit measures.

Primary efficacy endpoints included clinical global impression of change (CGI-C) judged by an independent experienced clinician—and a functional endpoint comprising the care–dependency subscale from a Dutch behavioral rating scale for geriatric patients (BGP), performed by experienced nursing staff.[7] Secondary efficacy variables included a modified D scale, a clinical global impression of severity of illness (CGI-S) and the BGP total score.[8,9] The D scale applied in the M-BEST study encompasses 16 functional variables characterizing the patient's independence within a wide range from normal functioning to total care dependence, and it is suitable for use by nurses.

Surprisingly, the independent observer reports showed a significant difference in favor of memantine compared with placebo from as early as 4 weeks of therapy. The difference was further increased after 3 months of treatment (Figure 9.1). The cumulative estimation of the coincidence of response in two independent variables, BGP and CGI-C, showed 61.3% coincidence of response in the memantine group and 47.4% coincidence of nonresponse in the placebo group, a finding which further supports a hypothesis of clinically meaningful improvement.

On the D scale, eight of the 16 measures showed significant improvement for memantine and these were significant for independent living, such as the ability to stand, move, and wash (Figure 9.2).

Practically speaking, these kinds of functional benefits are immensely helpful for the severe end of the dementia spectrum—not only to the patients and their families but also to the institutional carers, some of whom suffer from 'burnout' after extended periods working with profoundly demented patients.

The M-BEST study enrolled approximately equal numbers of AD and VaD sufferers. Memantine worked equally well in the two subpopulations stratified according to the Hachinski Ischemic Scale (HIS), showing equal response of 73% in both the HIS category of <5 and that of ≥ 5. The fact that the drug had an effect in both conditions suggests that severe dementia might be a common end stage for different diseases, although severe dementia itself cannot be considered to be a single disease entity.

Eighteen memantine patients (22%) and 18 placebo patients (21%) had adverse events, the most frequent of which was dizziness. Four memantine patients (5%) and five placebo patients (6%) experienced a serious adverse event, including myocardial infarctions and cerebrovascular accidents, all of which were rated by the investigators as unlikely to be related to the study medication.

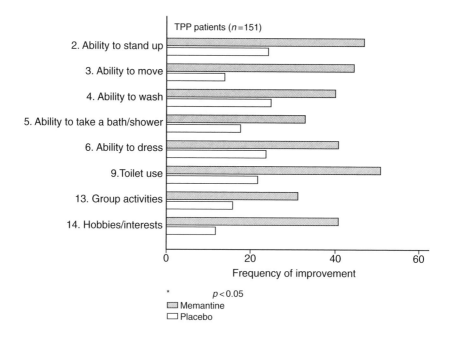

Figure 9.2

Functional endpoint results in M-Best

A randomized, placebo-controlled study of memantine, an uncompetitive NMDA antagonist, in patients with moderate to severe Alzheimer's disease

This study recruited 345 outpatients with severe AD (MMSE scores 3–14) at 32 centers in the USA, of which 252 were randomized. All patients met NINCDS–ADRDA criteria for AD.[10] The baseline characteristics of those randomized to the drug and placebo groups are summarized in Table 9.2.

The trial was designed as a randomized, two-arm, parallel-group study with patients taking either memantine (5 mg per day for 1 week, then 5 mg twice a day for 1 week, then 5 mg/10 mg per day for 1 week, and then 10 mg twice a day for the following 25 weeks) or placebo. Outcome measures included measures of cognition, function, and behavior, in keeping with guidelines from both European and US regulatory authorities.

The primary outcome measures were the Clinician's Interview-based Impression of Change plus Caregiver Input (CIBIC-Plus) global score[11] and change from baseline on the AD Cooperative Study Activities of Daily Living Inventory (ADCS-ADL)[12] modified for more severe dementia (ADCS-ADLsev).[13] Secondary outcome measures included a cognitive measure designed for patients with severe AD, the Severe Impairment Battery (SIB),[14,15] the MMSE, the Global Deterioration Scale (GDS),[16] the Functional Assessment Staging (FAST),[17] the Neuropsychiatric Inventory (NPI),[18] and the Resource Utilization in Dementia (RUD).[19]

At both endpoint (ITT) and week 28 (OC), change on the CIBIC-Plus favored memantine ($P = 0.06$, ITT; $P = 0.03$ OC). Memantine-treated patients deteriorated less than placebo-treated patients on the ADCSsev ($P = 0.02$, ITT; $P < 0.01$, OC), and these findings were consistent with the statistically significant benefits seen on the FAST. Cognition, as measured by the SIB,

Table 9.2. Severe AD study patient characteristics at (randomized patients, $n = 252$).

Characteristic	Placebo ($n = 126$)	Memantine (20 mg/day) ($n = 126$)	Total ($n = 252$)
Age, years ± SD	76.33 ± 7.76	75.94 ± 8.40	76.13 ± 8.07
Gender, n (%)			
Male	47 (37)	(35 (28)	82 (33)
Female	79 (63)	91 (72)	170 (67)
Severity of disease			
	8.05 ± 3.57	7.72 ± 3.72	7.88 ± 3.64
GDS stage 5, n (%)	53 (42)	59 (47)	112 (44)
GDS stage 6, n (%)	73 (58)	67 (53)	140 (56)

favored memantine ($P<0.001$, ITT; $P<0.01$, OC). Not surprisingly, the cognitive staging measures (MMSE and GDS) were not sensitive to the drug–placebo treatment differences, and there were no differences between those on drug and those on placebo on the NPI change score, but neuropsychiatric disorders were not highly prevalent in either group. Study results are summarized in Table 9.3.

The results of the RUD also favored memantine, with significantly less caregiver time needed to take care of those on drug versus those on placebo, and less overall costs associated with the care of memantine-treated patients.[5]

Most adverse events (AEs) in the study were mild to moderate and rated as either not related or unlikely to be related to the study drug. The incidence rates for the most frequently reported AEs and for those observed in more than 5% of the study population never exceeded the placebo rates by more than 2%. More placebo-treated patients left the study due to AEs than memantine-treated patients (17% versus 10%), and agitation, which was the most common AE leading to premature discontinuation, was more common in the placebo group.

Conclusions

NMDA receptor antagonists, such as memantine, may represent an important new alternative or addition to cholinergic therapy in the treatment of dementia. The evidence suggests that memantine therapy benefits both AD and VaD of moderate or severe degree, and studies are now underway in the USA to evaluate its use in mild to moderate AD. Clinical trials to date have been brief, and designed to show only symp-

Table 9.3. Severe AD study key efficacy results.

	LOCF analysis (last observation carried forward)			OC analysis (observed cases)		
	Memantine (n = 126)	Placebo (n = 126)	P-value*	Memantine (n = 97)	Placebo (n = 84)	P-value*
CIBIC-plus	4.52 (n = 118)	4.78 (n = 118)	0.0623	4.38	4.74	0.025
ADCS-ADL	−3.07 (n = 124)	−5.20 (n = 123)	0.0170	−2.49	−5.86	0.003
SIB	−3.99 (n = 124)	−10.08 (n = 123)	0.0002	−4.46	−10.16	0.002
FAST	0.21 (n = 121)	0.56 (n = 118)	0.0163	0.10	0.51	0.007

tomatic effects. Yet the mechanism of action (protection against excitotoxic neurodegeneration) suggests several theoretical points at which glutamatergic therapy may modify disease progression. In the future, suitably designed studies may confirm disease-modification benefits for dementia patients in the clinic. Meanwhile, it is apparent that short-term changes in rates of decline translate into cost benefits and benefits for caregivers seen as reduction in time spent caring for patients, as well as in dollars spent. If these benefits are sustained for even a few years, the savings to society and to individuals are substantial.

References

1. Winblad B, Poritis N. Memantine in severe dementia, results of the M-best study (benefit and efficacy in severely demented patients during treatment with memantine). Int J Geriatr Psychiatry 1999; 14:135–146.

2. Reisberg B, Doody R, Stoffler A et al. A randomized placebo controlled study of memantine, an uncompetitive NMDA antagonist, in patients with moderate to severe Alzheimer's disease. N Engl J Med 2003; 348:1333–1341.

3. Orgogozo JM, Rigaud A, Stoffler A et al. Efficacy of memantine in patients with mild to moderate vascular dementia: a randomized, placebo-controlled trial (MMM 300). Stroke 2002; 33:1834–1839.

4. Wilcock G, Möbius HJ, Stöffler A, on behalf of the MMM 500 group. A double-blind, placebo-controlled multicentre study of memantine in mild to moderate vascular dementia (MMM 500). Int Clin Psychopharmacol 2002; 17:297–305.

5. Wimo A, Winblad B, Stoffler A et al. Resource utilization and cost analysis of memantine in patients with moderate and severe Alzheimer's disease. Pharmacoeconomics 2003; 21:327–340.

6. Folstein M, Folstein S, McHugh P. Mini-mental state. A practical method for grading the cognitive state of patients for the clinician. J Psychiatr Res 1975; 12:189–198.

7. van der Kam P, Mol F, Wimmers MFHC. Beoordelingschaal voor oudere patienten (BGP). The Netherlands: Van Loghum Slaterus, 1971.

8. Ferm L. Behavioral activities in demented geriatric patients. Gerontol Clin 1974; 16:185–194.

9. van der Kam P, Hoeksma BH. The usefulness of BOP and SIVIS (ADL and behavior rating scales) for the estimation of workload in psychogeriatric nursing home. Results of a time-standard study. Tijdschr Gerontol Geriatr 1989; 20:159–166.

10. McKhann G, Drachman D, Folstein M et al. Clinical diagnosis of Alzheimer's disease: Report of the NINCDS–ADRDA Work Group Under the Auspices of the Department of Health and Human Services Task Force on Alzheimer's disease. Neurology 1984; 34:939–944.

11. Reisberg B, Schneider L, Doody R et al. Clinical global measures of dementia. Position paper from the International Working Group on Harmonization of Dementia Drug Guidelines. Alzheimer Dis Assoc Disord 1997; 11 (Suppl 3):8–18.

12. Galasko D, Bennett D, Sano M et al. An inventory to assess activities of daily living for clinical trials in Alzheimer's disease. The Alzheimer's Disease Cooperative Study, Alzheimer Dis Assoc Disord 1997; 11 (Suppl 2):S33–39.

13. Galasko D, Schmitt F, Jin S et al. Detailed assessment of cognition and activities of daily living in moderate and severe Alzheimer's disease. Neurobiol Aging 2000; 21 (Suppl 1);168 (Abstract).

14. Panisset M, Roudier M, Saxton J et al. Severe Impairment Battery: a neuropsychological test for severely demented patients. Arch Neurol 1994; 51:41–45.

15. Schmitt F, Ashford W, Ernesto C et al. The Severe Impairment Battery: concurrent validity and the assessment of longitudinal change in Alzheimer's disease. Alzheimer Dis Assoc Disord 1997; 11 (Suppl 2): S51–56.

16. Reisberg B, Ferris S, DeLeon M et al. Global deterioration scale for assessment of primary degenerative dementia. Am J Psychiatry 1982; 139:1136–1139.

17. Sclan S, Reisberg B. Functional assessment staging (FAST) in Alzheimer's disease; reliability, validity, and ordinality. Int Psychogeriatr 1992; 4 (Suppl 1):55–69.

18. Cummings J, Mega M, Gray K et al. The Neuropsychiatric Inventory: comprehensive assessment of psychopathology in dementia. Neurology 1994; 44: 2308–2314.

19. Wimo A, Wetterholm A, Mastey V et al. Evaluation of the healthcare resource utilization and caregiver time in anti-dementia drug trials. In: Wimo A, Jonsson B, Karlsson G, Winblad B, eds. Health Economics of Dementia. Chichester: Wiley, 1998; 465–499.

10
Management of comorbidity in Alzheimer's disease

Roy Jones

Introduction

Coexistent medical problems are very common in people with dementia. Most patients are elderly and are therefore likely to suffer from other illnesses, both acute and chronic. It is very important not to assume that every physical or mental problem a person with Alzheimer's disease (AD) experiences arises because of that disease.[1] Elderly people with dementia frequently have other therapeutically important medical conditions. One prospective study of 200 elderly outpatients with dementia identified 248 other medical diagnoses in 124 patients; 92 of the diagnoses were new.[2]

The existence of AD may require modification in the treatment of other medical conditions. This is increasingly being recognized as important. For example, a recent joint initiative from the Alzheimer's Association and the National Chronic Care Consortium in the USA is seeking to develop chronic care networks for people with AD and related dementias and their families. One of the goals is to define new clinical pathways in primary care to manage care across settings with new clinical guidelines for managing medical conditions and recognizing the comorbidity of AD and related dementia (www.nccconline.org/about/alzheimers.htm).

Coexistent medical problems require careful and skilled management. Other illnesses can increase the patient's confusion either temporarily or chronically. Drugs used to treat other conditions may themselves be responsible for worsening cognition. While other medical problems may have an adverse effect on the quality of life of patients and carers, their overzealous treatment, particularly at the end stage of AD, may be distressing as well.

Medical problems and their treatment can be aggravated by the inability of patients to report their own symptoms, so that regular review is essential. This becomes especially important when there has been acute deterioration in either cognition or behavior. Common conditions may present in an atypical or nonspecific manner. For example, there was a significant ($P < 0.001$) association between an impaired mental test score and atypical presentation of myocardial infarction.[3] It is also easy to overlook standard health measures, such as annual immunization against influenza and regular eye checks.

The purpose of the present chapter is to consider some of the commoner medical problems that are likely to be encountered and the practical relevance of these to the everyday management of the person with AD.

General health issues

Problems with hearing and vision

Older people often face communication difficulties because of poor hearing and vision. These difficulties are compounded in a person with memory problems where initial registration of information is even more critical. It is easy to overlook these problems, assuming that all of the difficulties are due to the dementia. All older people should have a regular test of hearing and vision (including the measurement of intraocular pressure to check for glaucoma), and this should be continued for as long as possible for a person with AD. It is important that the patient is accompanied to these examinations to ensure that the person carrying out the test is aware of the cognitive impairment. Some tests, such as examination of visual fields, may be difficult to carry out in patients with significant cognitive impairment, because of their failure to understand the requirements of the test.

There is limited research information about the occurrence of dementia and visual impairment. One study[4] reported impaired vision in 30 (28.8%) out of 114 community-resident people with dementia in comparison with 36 (34.6%) in a nondemented, age- and sex-matched control group. These differences were not significant. A study of vision impairment in nursing-home residents in Australia[5] concluded that residents with dementia had a slightly higher prevalence of blindness (13%) than those without dementia (9%). These results should be interpreted cautiously due to the small numbers in the study and the likelihood that blind people with dementia are more likely to need nursing home care.

Potential difficulties with vision and hearing must also be considered when testing memory and cognitive function. If the patient wears a hearing aid or reading glasses, then these should be used whenever they are being tested. This is not always easy when patients arrive at clinics, either without their reading glasses or having refused to wear their hearing aid. In our memory clinic, we always have spare pairs of reading glasses and a personal amplifying device with a stethoscope headset for use without a hearing aid. People with hearing problems prefer one-to-one conversations in a quiet room, because they find it more difficult to understand a conversation involving several people, especially in a noisy environment. Advice to the family may be of value in helping the AD patient with hearing problems to cope better in such situations.

Simple measures must not be overlooked. Sometimes the hearing problem merely requires removal of wax from the ears. Vision can often be improved by providing new glasses or by using brighter lighting.

Because people with AD frequently lose their glasses, it may seem useful to minimize the number of pairs of glasses that they possess or encourage them to wear them on a chain.[6] However, a recent study of more able older people living in community and retirement-village settings has suggested that multifocal (bifocal, trifocal, or progressive lens) glasses may impair edge-contrast sensitivity and depth perception, and increase the risk of falls in older people.[7] The conclusions of the study suggest that older people may benefit from wearing nonmultifocal glasses when negotiating stairs and in unfamiliar settings outside the home, and this may need to be borne in mind when considering the needs of people with AD.

Treatment of glaucoma is common in older people and important for the maintenance of good vision. Most medications used to treat glaucoma are in topical eyedrop form, and they can cause untoward systemic effects in older people. Side effects such as bradycardia from eyedrops containing the beta-blocker timolol may be particularly relevant in patients receiving cholinesterase inhibitors that can also potentially cause bradycardia. Clinicians must be aware of the untoward effects of these topical medications. It is also important that any medication review considers all medication including eyedrops.[8]

Foot problems

With age, numerous changes occur in the feet.[9] Foot disorders often cause discomfort and disability in older people. The ability to walk effectively and comfortably is important if one is to remain socially active. Degenerative changes in the feet can occur in a number of chronic diseases, such as diabetes mellitus with neuropathy, rheumatoid arthritis. and osteoarthritis. However, it is often simpler problems, such as curved or hypertrophied nails or fungal infections, that are troublesome, particularly in those who are perhaps unattentive to their own hygiene. When examining an older patient, it is important to inspect the feet, although patients may sometimes be reluctant to reveal what is under their socks or stockings. As with other older people, regular attention by a chiropodist can help, and this is particularly important in high-risk individuals, such as diabetics.

Dental problems

Dental hygiene and brushing to prevent gum and tooth disease may be performed inadequately by the patient with AD. Regular dental checkups are important, and this is true whether patients have their own teeth or dentures. Eating well is difficult without reasonable teeth, and ill-fitting dentures may impair both eating and speaking.

Too little attention is placed on oral hygiene and health in older people, particularly those unable to live independently, and residing in institutions and nursing homes.[10] A survey in the USA suggested that more than 25% of the population aged 65 and older had not seen a dental professional in the previous 5 years.[11] Moreover, older people who wore complete dentures were four times less likely to visit a dentist than those with remaining teeth. With improved oral health earlier in life, and greater retention of teeth, the dental needs of older people in the future will increase.[10] Dental care professionals recommend a number of procedures that will help maintain oral health in older people. For dentate individuals, these include oral hygiene after each meal with fluoridated toothpaste, toothbrushes, interproximal cleaners such as floss, and antimicrobial mouth rinses. These can reduce the risk of dental caries, periodontal infections, and halitosis. Edentate adults should use procedures such as denture cleansers and brushes.

A recent study suggests that simple measures such as twice-daily mastication for 15 min of a chewing gum containing xylitol and chlorhexidine can be implemented in older nursing-home residents to improve oral health.[12] This led to a reduction in angular cheilitis, denture stomatitis, and denture debris. The study involved close supervision and excluded the frailest patients in the nursing home, such as those with dementia. It may be difficult to get older people with AD to chew gum safely and effectively, so that it may not be possible to extrapolate these results. However, this study does suggest that dental hygiene may be improved by relatively simple measures, and that more attention should be paid to these issues by staff in residential and nursing facilities.

Nutrition, feeding problems, and weight loss

It is easy to forget the important link between good nutrition and general health and well-being in those with dementia, especially if they live alone. People with dementia are often underweight and have feeding problems (for example, see Sandman et al[13]). Weight loss has been considered almost inevitable in people with AD and other dementias. However, this is not always the case.[14,15] Some patients with AD actually overeat and may indulge in bingeing.[16]

Undernutrition may contribute to other conditions such as muscle and weight loss, constipation, and anemia. A person with AD must be encouraged and, if necessary, helped to eat nutritious, balanced meals. Patients can often be helped through common sense and creativity—for example, providing ready access to snacks and drinks, feeding patients at times during the day when they are at their best, and considering any food fads that they may have.

For a more detailed discussion of nutrition in dementia, see Chapter 11.

Urinary incontinence

Urinary incontinence in dementia is not always due to dementia. Urinary incontinence is unfortunately a common problem that is increasingly prevalent in older people. A community prevalence study found a prevalence of 6% in the over-65s and 15% in the over-85s (both sexes).[17] A census of urinary incontinence in Leicestershire, UK, reported that about two-thirds of people in private nursing homes were incontinent of urine, compared with one-third in residential homes.[18] There is a substantial overlap between urinary incontinence and physical dependency, as well as with impaired cognitive function.[19] In a study of institutionalized patients in Italy, 36.2% of those with good cognitive function had urinary tract incontinence, in comparison with 76.7% of demented subjects. Although incontinence is common in patients with AD it is not inevitable; unfortunately, it may be somewhat neglected, affecting the quality of life not only of the sufferer but especially of the carer. Indeed, urinary (and especially fecal) incontinence may play an important part in the decision to institutionalize a person with AD.[20,21] Urinary incontinence is also very expensive, costing the UK National Health Service about £70 million a year in aids and appliances.[22]

Unfortunately, there have been very few randomized, controlled trials of interventions for incontinence in the presence of dementia. It is essential to try to assess the nature and cause of the problem, including urgency and frequency. A physical examination (including rectal and vaginal examinations) is necessary, together with appropriate investigations. The urine must be examined, even if obtaining a proper midstream sample is difficult. A urinary tract infection is a common problem in older people and may lead to incontinence, as may the use of diuretic therapy. Requirements for maintaining continence are shown in Table 10.1.[23] These requirements may be particularly difficult for a patient with dementia who is physically immobile or slow, or in an unfamiliar place and uncertain where the toilet is. Leaving a night light on may help patients that tend to get lost indoors.

The treatment of urinary incontinence may be based on Good Clinical Practice consensus guidelines.[24] Management should involve the multidisciplinary team. A number of general measures can be taken, including controlling fluid and caffeine consumption, as well as dealing with constipation. If infection and constipation have been excluded, developing a program of regular toileting that matches the patient's own voiding pattern can help.[25] Cautious use of drugs such as tolterodine and oxybutynin may be of value, although the evidence for this is not clear.[26,27] There are also concerns that oxybutynin itself can cause cognitive impairment in older individuals, consis-

Table 10.1. Abilities needed to maintain continence.[23]

Appreciation of the need to void
Ability to alert a caregiver (if necessary)
Adequate motivation
Adequate mobility (to reach the toilet, transfer to a commode, or use an appliance)
Awareness of the appropriate time and place to void
Ability to initiate voluntary voiding

tent with the known cognitive effects of anticholinergic medication.[28] Great care is therefore needed in the use of such drugs, and they should be administered at the lowest dose possible. It has been suggested that behavioral strategies are more likely to be beneficial than drug treatment for older people with urinary incontinence in nursing homes.[19] Such strategies include timed voiding, habit retraining, and prompted voiding. Prompted voiding is a behavioral strategy for which there is the most supportive evidence.[19] This strategy encourages people to initiate their own toileting through requests for help and positive reinforcement from carers when they do this. The degree of cognitive impairment of subjects does not seem to be helpful in predicting response to a prompted voiding program,[29] although it is likely that this approach will be difficult for patients with severe dementia.[19]

Fecal incontinence and constipation

Fecal incontinence, while less common than urinary incontinence, is undoubtedly more embarrassing and distressing to both patient and carers. It should be afforded a higher priority[30] and has a major influence on institutionalization. Like urinary incontinence, fecal incontinence should not be regarded as normal in demented patients and can be managed, improved, or sometimes cured.[31] There is very little published research on fecal incontinence in dementia. It can arise when the normal reaction to the sensation of a full rectum is lost. It can also arise in response to diarrhea from any cause (including as a side effect of cholinesterase inhibitors). If an underlying cause can be discovered, it should obviously be treated. Nonspecific diarrhea may respond to bulking agents and antidiarrheal drugs. Sometimes regular enemas will be necessary to clear the bowel.

Somewhat as a contradiction, constipation can also lead to both fecal and urinary incontinence. The frequency of constipation increases with age. It can also be exacerbated by drugs such as opioid analgesics, iron supplements, diuretics, or aluminum-containing antacids (magnesium-containing antacids tend to cause diarrhea). Other factors already discussed elsewhere in this chapter, such as immobility and inadequate diet, may also aggravate the situation in people with AD. If constipation is severe or causes fecal impaction, secondary diarrhea and overflow fecal incontinence can occur, as can urinary incontinence. Although laxatives and enemas may be necessary, at least initially, increasing fluid and fiber intake may provide a more lasting solution.

Falls and fractures

Patients with AD are at increased risk of falls and fractures, particularly of the neck of the femur and these are associated with admission to long-term care.[32,33] A study of the epidemiology of injury in people with AD showed that the risk of injury is related to disease severity.[34] However, risk of injury tends to decline in very severe dementia, probably due to immobility and reduced activity. Falls in people with dementia are more likely to result in fracture than in elderly people in general.[34]

The psychological consequences of falling may be significant particularly in patients with AD who already have reduced self-confidence. This can lead to a vicious circle of restricted activity, increased dependence, and reduced mobility, followed by further falls, eventually leading to patients moving to a more supervised environment.[35] It is important to consider why people are falling and, as with other conditions in people with dementia, not to assume it is merely a result of dementia. Falls can arise from a medical condition such as postural hypotension, problems with vision and balance, drugs, agitation, and environmental hazards. In addition, patients with AD may have poor judgment, poor concentration to avoid environmental hazards, and disturbances of gait. Psychotropic medication may certainly increase the risk of falls;[36] and there have also been suggestions that cholinesterase inhibitors might potentially increase the risk of falling, possibly as a result of the bradycardia that these drugs cause.[37] The recent guidelines for prevention of falls in older people[36] are helpful and should be read by those working with people with dementia. Reducing psychotropic medication is of benefit, and hip protectors may protect those at highest risk from hip fractures.[36]

Management of pain

People with significant cognitive impairment, such as AD, may not be able to explain satisfactorily that they are in pain,[38] even though this may significantly reduce their ability to function normally. Acute pain due to retention of urine, a fracture, or some other cause may be noted only as a change in behavior, agitation, or increasing confusion. It has been suggested that one of the behavioral symptoms associated with physical discomfort is 'verbal outburst',[39] but another study found that verbally disruptive behavior was no more likely in subjects with pain than those without.[40] Clinicians need to be aware of this when assessing any recent change in activity or behavior. Table 10.2 lists some of the verbal and nonverbal pain-related behaviors and changes in normal functioning that may be seen.[41]

Painful conditions are both underdetected and undertreated in people with dementia living in institutions.[38] In nursing homes and other settings, they are less likely to be prescribed analgesics than cognitively intact residents.[40,42] Assessing pain in residents with dementia challenges the assessor because the process involves much uncertainty.[43] Older people with dementia must be encouraged to report their pain and these reports should be trusted (for example, see Hurley et al[44] and Ferrell et al[45]). Yet, very often, the only assessment possible is based on caregivers' perceptions through direct observation, which may or may not be accurate.[46,47] A study of cognitively impaired nursing-home residents validated the geriatrician's evaluations of pain during a medical examination for moderately impaired people, but not in the severely cognitively impaired.[43]

Table 10.2. Common pain behaviors in cognitively impaired elderly people.[41]

Facial expressions
  Slight frown; sad, frightened face
  Grimacing; wrinkled forehead; closed or tightened eyes
  Any distorted expression
  Rapid blinking

Verbalizations, vocalizations
  Sighing, moaning, groaning
  Grunting, chanting, calling out
  Noisy breathing
  Asking for help
  Verbally abusive

Body movements
  Rigid, tense body posture; guarding
  Fidgeting
  Increased pacing; rocking
  Restricted movement
  Gait or mobility changes

Changes in interpersonal interaction
  Aggressive, combative, resisting care
  Decreased social interactions
  Socially inappropriate, disruptive
  Withdrawn

Changes in activity patterns or routines
  Refusing food; appetite change
  Increase in rest periods
  Sleep, rest pattern changes
  Sudden cessation of common routines
  Increased wandering

Mental status changes
  Crying or tears
  Increased confusion
  Irritability or distress

Note: some patients demonstrate little or no specific behavior associated with severe pain.

In any assessment, the most obvious causes of pain must be excluded. In the absence of a diagnosis and if pain is suspected, a therapeutic trial of an analgesic is the only reasonable approach. Better methods for assessment of pain in severe dementia are also needed, and several research teams are investigating this.[43] When selecting an analgesic, the least toxic means of achieving systemic pain relief should be used. For managing persistent pain in older people, an American Geriatrics Society panel has recently published recommendations.[41] Paracetamol (acetaminophen) should be the first drug to consider in the treatment of mild to moderate pain of musculoskeletal origin. Traditional (nonselective) NSAIDs should be avoided in treating patients who require long-term, daily analgesic therapy. The COX-2 selective agents, or nonacetylated salicylates, are preferred for older people who require NSAIDs. Opioid analgesic drugs may help relieve moderate to severe pain. They should be used on an 'as-needed' basis for episodic pain, but long-acting or sustained-release analgesic preparations are suggested for continuous pain. Fixed-dose combinations of opioid with paracetamol or NSAIDs may be useful for mild to moderate pain.

The guidelines also emphasize the prevention of problems such as opioid-related constipation, sedation, and impaired cognitive performance, and these are especially relevant in patients with AD. As with all medication in patients with AD, the situation should be re-evaluated frequently for both efficacy and side effects, including symptoms or signs of gastrointestinal blood loss in patients on long-term NSAIDs.

Terminal care

Patients in the latter stages of AD are likely to be immobile, doubly incontinent, and mute. They may require feeding and need to be turned to avoid pressure sores. At this stage, patients are likely to die as a result of dehydration, aspiration pneumonia, and sepsis, although they may also succumb to disorders that may affect all older people, such as stroke and cancer. One study has suggested that age, sex, functional limitation, and malnutrition are the strongest predictors of death for AD patients in nursing homes.[48]

When people with dementia reach the terminal phase of their illness, they require effective palliative care just like patients with physical conditions. Their families also need counseling and support. There is evidence that these needs are not being met.[49] In the last year of their life, patients with dementia are seen less often than cancer patients, and their carers rated the help they receive from general practitioners less highly. Patients dying from dementia appear to have similar health care needs and symptoms (confusion, incontinence, pain, low mood, constipation, and loss of appetite). The principles of terminal care developed by the hospice movement must be applied to patients with AD and other dementias, whose limited cooperation demands extra skill and empathy from everyone who looks after them.

In the terminal stages of the disease, it is also important to recognize when further active treatment is doing more harm than good. One example of this is tube feeding, which appears to be more common in the USA than in the UK, where it is relatively uncommon. Even setting aside the ethical considerations, it is unclear that tube feeding improves any clinically relevant outcomes, such as preventing aspiration pneumonia or reducing the risk of infection or pressure sores. Some evidence suggests that it may even worsen outcomes.[50]

A recent study in the UK has examined the attitudes of carers and old-age psychiatrists towards the treatment of potentially fatal events in end-stage dementia.[51] The ethical issues involved in end-of-life decisions are especially difficult when patients have lost the capacity to express their wishes about treatments. In general, doctors, working with carers, make these decisions on behalf of the patient. In this study, 148 carers and 34 old-age psychiatrists responded to an attitudinal questionnaire. There were significant differences between carers' and clinicians' attitudes. Clinicians were less likely to favor active treatment of potentially fatal events than carers. However, carers also valued patient-centered issues, such as dying with dignity, the patient's best interests, and the patient's wishes more than the clinicians. Such differences may affect decision making. Considerably more clinician/carer debate and dialogue seems to be needed,[51] and this at a time when legislation proposed for England will involve carers more formally in such decisions.[52,53]

Specific medical conditions

The previous part of this chapter has considered general health issues that create problems for patients with AD, their families, and the multidisciplinary team that is involved with their care. There are a number of more specific medical conditions that are likely to be important in the patient with AD and worthy of particular mention. They are common conditions in elderly people and responsible for ill health even in the absence of dementia, although they may usually be considered to be more commonly associated with vascular dementia. For a more detailed discussion of these conditions, see Chapter 2.

Diabetes mellitus

The management of diabetes mellitus, whether recent or long-standing, may be particularly challenging in the patient with AD and impaired cognition. Ideally, the management of diabetes depends on a cooperative and adequately informed patient. Poorly controlled diabetes may lead to further cognitive damage and other problems. But, while good control of the blood-sugar level may reduce the rate of intellectual decline, it is very important to minimize the risk of hypoglycemia. In general, therefore, it is usually safer to aim for only moderately good control of the blood sugar.

It is preferable that newly diagnosed non-insulin-dependent diabetics be given at least 3 months' dietary restriction and encouraged to increase their physical activity. This may not be practical for people with AD, especially if they are elderly. The risk of hypoglycemic episodes from long-acting sulfonylureas is greater in older individuals. It is therefore preferable to avoid chlorpropamide and probably glibencamide. These may be replaced by drugs such as gliclazide, glipizide, and tolbutamide, which must be given in divided doses. Insulin is best avoided if possible.

Hypertension

Despite good evidence for the effectiveness of treating hypertension in older people, clinicians are often reluctant to do so. Asymptomatic hypertension can be a particular dilemma in an elderly person with AD. There may be concerns about compliance and also the risk from side effects, particularly postural hypotension.

Successful blood pressure control can enhance cognitive performance, at least in patients with multiinfarct dementia.[54] Antihypertensive treatment is also associated with a lower incidence of dementia in elderly people with isolated systolic hypertension.[55] However, it may be unreasonable to treat hypertension too aggressively, particularly in patients with severe dementia.

In general, it is appropriate to treat hypertension conventionally in patients with AD. Therapy should be initiated with a low dose of a thiazide diuretic such as bendrofluazide, 2.5 mg daily, following which a low dose of a beta-blocker such as atenolol, 25 mg daily, can be added if there are no contraindications. Beta-blockers can occasionally cause confusion. Diabetic patients and those who cannot tolerate beta-blockers are better managed with an angiotensin-converting enzyme inhibitor. Information regarding calcium-channel blockers is contradictory. There are data to suggest that they are associated with a lower incidence of dementia,[55] while another study suggested they were more likely to be associated with cognitive decline.[56]

Atrial fibrillation

Atrial fibrillation (AF) affects 5% of those over 65 and 10% of those over 75.[57] Guidelines concerning the management of permanent AF are clear in their recommendation of the use of anticoagulant and antiplatelet drugs that can reduce the risk of stroke.

There is a fivefold increase in stroke risk (to approximately 5% per year). The risk of stroke appears to be reduced by about two-thirds with warfarin and by about one-fifth with aspirin. The highest risk is seen in people with a previous stroke, those over the age of 75, and those with hypertension, coronary artery disease, diabetes, heart failure, or left ventricular dysfunction.[57]

Studies confirm that older patients with AF have the lowest frequency of anticoagulant use.[58] Dementia also appears to be a significant independent determinant of nontreatment with aspirin or warfarin when otherwise indicated for the prevention of recurrent stroke.[58]

The underutilization of aspirin and warfarin in older stroke patients with dementia may be a modifiable basis for their increased risk of recurrence and death.[58] However, there is an understandable reluctance to use warfarin in people with a condition like AD where compliance is likely to be a problem.

Clearly, the clinician must take into account a patient's overall situation in trying to decide whether the benefits of anticoagulation outweigh any risks.

In many cases, the less effective but usually safer alternative of aspirin, 75–300 mg/day, or an alternative antiplatelet drug, such as clopidogrel, will be selected.

Medication

Drug therapy undoubtedly brings great benefits to the quality of life for many older people, but the adverse effects of drugs can lead to serious problems and misery. The use of drug therapy in AD requires even greater considera- tion. Many drugs can increase cognitive impairment, and this may be misinterpreted as a deterioration in the underlying AD. Sedation, postural hypotension, and falls are other nonspecific adverse effects that may be caused by drug therapy.

The list of drugs that may theoretically cause confusion is large, but it is especially likely with drugs that have anticholinergic properties. Such drugs may cause acute or more chronic confusion; the more commonly used drugs that can cause confusion are shown in Table 10.3. Clinicians should always be careful when introducing any new drug to a patient with AD, but

Table 10.3. Drugs causing acute confusion.[1]

Drugs with anticholinergic properties
    Antihistamines (such as diphenhydramine)
    Antispasmodics
    Tricyclic antidepressants
    Antipsychotics
    Antiparkinsonian drugs
    Oxybutynin

Other drugs
    Benzodiazepines
    Alcohol
    Trazodone and other antidepressants
    Narcotic analgesics
    Lithium carbonate
    Digoxin
    Diuretics
    Antihypertensives (?especially calcium-channel blockers)
    Anticonvulsants
    Cimetidine
    Steroids
    Indomethacin and other nonsteroidals

Drug withdrawal
    Alcohol
    Benzodiazepines

the drugs in the list require particular care. If a patient has become acutely confused, any recent changes in drug therapy must always be considered as a possible cause. All drug therapy for patients with AD should be reviewed regularly; for example, diuretics may produce electrolyte imbalance, and this can cause confusion at any time, especially if the patient develops other problems such as diarrhea.

Standard doses of drugs should also be reconsidered with increasing age. There is an inevitable decline in renal and hepatic reserves with increasing age and weight loss is also common. Doses of drugs for conditions such as epilepsy or hypertension that were satisfactory in former years may be too large for the frailer, older patient with AD.

There is a particular risk with neuroleptic and other drugs that are used to control behavioral problems in the patient with AD. These drugs may have nonspecific effects, such as sedation, which can lead to immobility, incontinence, and other problems. It has also been suggested that neuroleptics may hasten cognitive decline.[59]

Acknowledgments

I thank Maggie Hawkes and Lesley Jones for their secretarial help.

References

1. Jones RW. Drug Treatment in Dementia. Oxford: Blackwell Science, 2000.

2. Larson EB, Reifler BV, Sumi SM et al. Diagnostic tests in the evaluation of dementia; a prospective study of 200 elderly outpatients. Arch Intern Med 1986; 146:1917–1922.

3. Black DA. Mental state and presentation of myocardial infarction in the elderly. Age Ageing 1987; 16:125–127.

4. Philp I, McKee KJ, Meldrum P et al. Community care of demented and non-demented elderly people: a comparison study of financial burden, service use, and unmet needs in family supporters. BMJ 1995; 310:1503–1505.

5. Mitchell P, Hayes P, Wang J. Visual impairment in nursing home residents: the Blue Mountains Eye Study. Med J Aust 1997; 166:73–76.

6. Mace NL, Rabins PV. The 36-Hour Day, 3rd edn. Baltimore MD: Johns Hopkins University Press, 1999.

7. Lord SR, Dayhew J, Howland A. Multifocal glasses impair H-contrast sensitivity and depth perception and increase the risk of falls in older people. J Am Geriatr Soc 2002; 50:1760–1766.

8. Novack GD, O'Donnell MJ, Molloy DW. New glaucoma medications in the geriatric population: efficacy and safety. J Am Geriatr Soc 2002; 50:956–962.

9. Helfand AE. Foot problems. In: Evans JG, Williams PF, Michel J-P, Beattie L, eds. Oxford Textbook of Geriatric Medicine, 2nd edn.

Oxford: Oxford University Press, 2000:602–613.

10. Ship JA. Improving oral health in older people. J Am Geriatr Soc 2002; 50:1454–1455.

11. Gift HC, Newman JF. How older adults use oral health care services: results of a National Health Interview Survey. J Am Dent Assoc 1993; 124:89–93.

12. Simons D, Brailsford SR, Kidd EAN, Beighton D. The effect of medicated chewing gums on oral health in frail older people: a one-year clinical trial. J Am Geriatr Soc 2002; 50:1348–1353.

13. Sandman TO, Adolfsson R, Nygren C et al. Nutritional status and dietary intake in institutionalised patients with Alzheimer's disease and multi-infarct dementia. J Am Geriatr Soc 1987; 35:31–38.

14. Franzoni S, Frisoni GB, Boffelli S et al. Good nutritional oral intake is associated with equal survival in demented and nondemented very old patients. J Am Geriatr Soc 1996; 44:1366–1370.

15. Wang SY, Sukagawa N, Hossain M, Ooi WL. Longitudinal weight changes, length of survival and energy requirements of long-term care residents with dementia. J Am Geriatr Soc 1997; 45:1189–1195.

16. Hope T, Keene J. Behavioural problems in dementia and biochemistry: clinical aspects. Neurodegeneration 1996; 5:399–402.

17. McGrother CW, Castleden CM, Duffin HM et al. A profile of disordered micturition in the elderly at home. Age Ageing 1987; 16:105–110.

18. Peet SM, Castleden CM, McGrother CW. Prevalence of urinary and fecal incontinence in hospitals, residential and nursing homes for older people. BMJ 1995; 311:1062–1064.

19. Durrant J, Snape J. Urinary incontinence in nursing homes for older people. Age Ageing 2003; 32:12–18.

20. Ouslander JG, Zarit SH, Orr NK, Muira SA. Incontinence among elderly community-dwelling dementia patients. Characteristics, management, and impact on caregivers. J Am Geriatr Soc 1990; 38:440–445.

21. O'Donnell BF, Drachman DA, Barnes HJ et al. Incontinence and troublesome behaviour predict institutionalisation in dementia. J Geriatr Psychiatry Neurol 1992; 5:45–52.

22. O'Brien J, Long H. Urinary incontinence: long-term effectiveness of nursing intervention in primary care. BMJ 1995; 311:1208.

23. Smith N, Clamp M, Neurological causes of incontinence. In: Continence Promotion in General Practice. Oxford: Oxford University Press, 1991: 38–40.

24. Urinary Incontinence Guidelines Panel. Urinary incontinence in Adults, Clinical Practice Guidelines. AHCPR Publication No. 92-0038. Rockville MD: Agency for Health Care Policy, 1992.

25. Jirovec NN. Urine control in patients with chronic degenerative brain disease. In: Ortman HJ, ed. Alzheimer's Disease: Problems, Prospects and Perspectives. New York: Plenum Press, 1986.

26. Castleden CM, Duffin HM, Gulati RS. Double blind study of imipramine and placebo for incontinence due to bladder instability. Age Ageing 1986; 15:299–303.

27. Ouslander JG, Schnelle JF, Uman G et al. Does oxybutynin add to the effectiveness of prompted voiding for urinary incontinence among nursing home residents? A placebo controlled trial. J Am Geriatr Soc 1995; 43:610–617.

28. Katz IR, Sands LP, Bilker W et al. Identification of medications that cause cognitive impairment in older people: the case of oxybutynin chloride. J Am Geriatr Soc 1998; 46:8–13.

29. Ouslander JG, Schnelle JF, Uman G et al. Predictors of successful prompted voiding among incontinent nursing home residents. JAMA 1995; 273:1366–1370.

30. Crome P. Prevalence of faecal incontinence. Age Ageing 2002; 31:322.

31. Resnick N, Ouslander JG. Urinary incontinence—where do we stand and where do we go from here? J Am Geriatr Soc 1990; 38:263–264.

32. McLennan WJ, Isles FE. Medical and social factors influencing admission to residential care. BMJ 1984; 288:701–703.

33. Sattin RW. Falls among older persons: public health perspective. Annu Rev Publ Health 1992; 13:489–508.

34. Oleske DN, Wilson RS, Bernard BA et al. Epidemiology of injury in people with Alzheimer's disease. J Am Geriatr Soc 1995; 43:741–746.

35. Tinettin E, Powell L. Fear of falling and low self-efficacy: a cause of dependence in elderly persons. J Gerontol 1993; 48 (Special Issue):35–38.

36. American Geriatrics Society, British Geriatrics Society, and American Academy of Orthopedic Surgeons Panel on Falls Prevention. Guideline for the prevention of falls in older persons. J Am Geriatr Soc 2001; 49:664–672.

37. Schneider LS. Treatment of Alzheimer's disease with cholinesterase inhibitors. Clin Geriatr Med 2001; 17:337–358.

38. Cook AKR, Niven CA, Downs MG. Assessing the pain of people with cognitive impairment. Int J Geriatr Psychiatry 1999; 14:421–425.

39. Kovach CR, Weissman DE, Griffie J et al. Assessment and treatment of discomforts for people with late-stage dementia. J Pain Symptom Manage 1999; 18:412–419.

40. Brummel-Smith K, London MR, Drew N et al. Outcomes of pain in frail older adults with dementia. J Am Geriatr Soc 2002; 50:1847–1851.

41. AGS Panel on Persistent Pain in Older Persons. The management of persistent pain in older persons. J Am Geriatr Soc 2002; 50:S205-S224.

42. Scherder EJ. Low use of analgesics in Alzheimer's disease: possible mechanisms. Psychiatry 2000; 63:1–12.

43. Cohen-Mansfield J, Lipson S. Pain in cognitively impaired nursing home residents; how well are physicians diagnosing it? J Am Geriatr Soc 2002; 50:1039–1044.

44. Hurley AC, Volicer BJ, Hanrahan TA et al. Assessment of discomfort in advanced Alzheimer's patients. Res Nurs Health 1992; 15:369–377.

45. Ferrell BA, Ferrell BR, Rivera L. Pain in cognitively impaired nursing home patients. J Pain Symptom Manage 1995; 10:591–598.

46. Galloway S, Turner L. Pain assessment in older adults who are

cognitively impaired. J Gerontol Nurs 1999; 25:34–39.

47. Weiner D, Peterson B, Keefe F. Chronic pain-associated behaviors in the nursing home: resident versus care-giver perceptions. Pain 1999; 80:577–588.

48. Gambassi G, Landi F, Lapane KL et al. Predictors of mortality in patients with Alzheimer's disease living in nursing homes. J Neurol Neurosurg Psychiatry 1999; 67:59–65.

49. McCarthy M, Addington-Hall J, Altmann D. The experience of dying with dementia: a retrospective study. Int J Geriatr Psychiatry 1997; 12:404–409.

50. Finucane TE, Christmas C, Travis K. Tube feeding in patients with advanced dementia; a review of the evidence. J Am Med Assoc 1999; 282:1365–1370.

51. Coetzee RH, Leask SJ, Jones RG. The attitudes of carers and old age psychiatrists towards the treatment of potentially fatal events in end-stage dementia. Int J Geriatr Psychiatry 2003; 18:169–173.

52. The Law Commission. Mental Incapacity—Item 9 of the Fourth Programme of Law Reform: Mentally Incapacitated Adults. Law Commission LAW COM 1995; 231:189–212.

53. The Lord High Chancellor. 'Making Decisions': the Government's proposals for making decisions on behalf of mentally incapacitated adults, presented to Parliament by the Lord High Chancellor by Command of Her Majesty (Cm 4465), 1999.

54. Meyer JS, Judd BW, Tawaklna T et al. Improved cognition after control of risk factors for multi-infarct dementia. JAMA 1986; 256:2203–2209.

55. Forette F, Seux M-L, Staessen JA et al. Prevention of dementia in randomised double-blind placebo-controlled Systolic Hypertension in Europe (Syst-Eur) trial. Lancet 1998; 352:1347–1351.

56. Dinsdale H. Searching for a link between calcium-channel blockers and cognitive function. Can Med Assoc J 1999; 161:534–535.

57. Hampton JR. The management of atrial fibrillation in elderly patients. Age Ageing 1999; 28:249–250.

58. Moroney JT, Tseng C-L, Paik MC et al. Treatment for the secondary prevention of stroke in older patients; the influence of dementia status. J Am Geriatr Soc 1999; 47:824-829.

59. McShane R, Keene J, Gedling K et al. Do neuroleptic drugs hasten cognitive decline in dementia? Prospective study with necropsy follow-up. BMJ 1997; 314:266–270.

11
Nutritional prevention in Alzheimer's disease: The prospect for the future?

Olivier Guerin and Bruno Vellas

Introduction

Alzheimer's disease (AD) begins to manifest itself by memory deficits and difficulty in abstract thinking. As the brain lesions spread, the cognitive deficits progressively worsen and problems of orientation and behavior, loss of autonomy, and eating disorder appear. Weight loss is a nutritional problem frequently observed in patients with dementia of Alzheimer type, as demonstrated in clinical practice and in numerous studies. But nutritional problems should not, perhaps, be seen only as a consequence of this disease: in fact, nutrition seems to influence cognitive function and behavior. Numerous works have reported an association between alterations in cognitive function and vitamin status (principally, the B group vitamins and the products involved in their metabolism, and the antioxidant vitamins), consumption of cholesterol and fatty acids, and overall energy intake. Table 11.1 summarizes the most significant studies published in 2002.

A continuum

Dementia of Alzheimer type is being diagnosed earlier and earlier, thanks to more numerous memory clinics, the increasing precision of neuropsychological evaluation, and the growing interest of treating physicians, who are now well informed.

There are several nosological frameworks to define the cognitive and particularly the memory deficits of the elderly subject, especially those at the borderline of the abnormal (one or two standard deviations on the tests). The most commonly used is mild cognitive impairment (MCI). This is an objective cognitive deficit with a memory or attention complaint which is within normal range and has no functional impact on daily life. Prospective studies have shown that each year 12–15% of these patients progress to AD.

Numerous ongoing studies are attempting to identify which patients with MCI are at risk of developing AD and to recognize the early forms.

Table 11.1. Most important studies of the year 2002 on nutritional prevention in Alzheimer's disease.

Study	Subjects	Findings
Johnson-Kozlow et al[30]	1037 subj. (mean age 73 years)	Higher lifetime coffee consumption in women was associated with better cognitive performance.
Truelsen et al[18]	1709 subj. (>65 years)	Average weekly total alcohol intake had no significant effect on risk of dementia. Monthly and weekly intake of wine was significantly associated with a lower risk of dementia.
Ruitenberg et al[17]	7983 subj. (>55 years)	Light-to-moderate drinking (one to three drinks per day) was significantly associated with a lower risk of any dementia. The effect seems to be unchanged by the source of alcohol.
Engelhart et al[15]	5395 subj. (>55 years)	High dietary intake of vitamins C and E may lower the risk of AD.
Morris et al[13]	2889 subj. (mean age 74 years)	Vitamin E intake, from foods or supplements, is associated with less cognitive decline with age.
Morris et al[14]	815 subj. (>65 years)	This study suggests that vitamin E from food, but not other antioxidants, may be associated with a reduced risk of AD. Unexpectedly, this association was observed only among individuals without the ApoE4 allele.
Prins et al[28]	1077 subj. (aged 60–90 years)	Elevated plasma total homocysteine levels are associated with decreased cognitive performance in nondemented elderly people, and the relation was most marked for psychomotor speed.
Seshadri et al[25]	1092 subj. (mean age 76 years)	Increased plasma homocysteine level is a strong, independent risk factor for the development of dementia and AD.
Yaffe et al[20]	1037 women (mean age 71 years)	High LDL and total cholesterol levels are associated with cognitive impairment, and lowering these lipoprotein levels may be a strategy for preventing impairment.
Kivipelto et al[19]	1449 subj. (>65 years)	The ApoE4 allele, elevated midlife total cholesterol level, and high midlife systolic blood pressure are independent risk factors for AD. The risk of AD from treatable factors appears to be greater than that from the ApoE4 allele.
Luchsinger et al[2]	980 subj. (mean age 75.3 years)	Higher intake of calories and fats may be associated with higher risk of AD in individuals carrying the ApoE4 allele.

Moreover, recent studies have shown that subjects aged over 75 years who seek medical advice for a memory complaint are at greater risk of developing AD. A continuum between cognitive complaints, MCI, and AD does therefore seem to exist.

In fact, it will be more than 10 years before the pathophysiological mechanisms give rise to clinical signs. There is therefore time to plan preventive strategies; among these, nutrition is attracting particular attention at the present time.

The theory underlying research on nutrition and AD relates to free radicals. Peroxidation of membrane polyunsaturated fatty acids (PUFA) following damage by free radicals could be involved in brain deterioration and cause alteration of enzyme activity, transport functions, and receptor–ligand interaction, and loss of membrane lipid bilayer asymmetry and thus of membrane fluidity. Such changes may alter ion channels and neurotransmitter transport, and thus be an underlying cause of brain dysfunction.

Another element which may open the possibility of prevention through nutrition is the vascular determinant. In fact, AD and vascular lesions are found in association more frequently than would be the case by chance. The brains of nondemented patients who had died of coronary diseases were found to contain more senile plaques than those of patients who had died of other causes.[1] The most recent works implicate homocysteine as a probable risk factor for AD through microvascular lesions. In addition, arterial hypertension, diabetes and hypercholesterolemia are factors not only of vascular dementia, but also of AD.

The present study will consider first of all the links between oxidative stress, nutrition, and AD, and then those between vascular risk factors, nutrition, and AD, bearing in mind that these two processes are also linked.

The role of oxidative stress

Oxidative stress, calorie intake, and fatty acids

In numerous animal models, life expectancy has been found to be significantly higher in groups with reduced calorie intake compared with control groups fed ad libitum. Some teams thus raised the question of a possible association between calorie intake and AD.

Luchsinger et al[2] followed 980 elderly persons (mean age 75.3 years, 67% women) for a mean of 4 years. Data on total daily calorie intake and carbohydrate, protein, and fat intakes were collected by a semiquantitative food-frequency questionnaire. Twenty-eight percent of subjects were homo- or heterozygous for the apolipoprotein E epsilon4 allele (ApoE4). During the follow-up, 242 cases of AD were diagnosed (an annual incidence of 6%). Patients whose calorie intake was in the highest quartile had a greater risk of AD than patients whose intake was in the lowest quartile (OR 1.5; CI 1.0,

2.2). In ApoE4 subjects, the odds ratio was 2.3 (CI 1.1, 4.7). In the population as a whole, fat intake did not appear to be a significant risk factor. In ApoE4 patients, however, fat intake was a risk factor for AD, with an odds ratio of 2.3 (CI 1.1, 4.9) for the highest quartile group compared with the lowest quartile group.

Otsuka et al[3] studied nutritional intake in subjects with AD (27 patients), subjects with vascular dementia (15 patients), and 49 age-matched controls. The two patient groups had a higher energy intake than the controls: +25% for patients with AD; +35% for those with vascular dementia. In both these groups, the men had a higher intake of n-6 PUFA and the women a lower intake of n-3 PUFA than the control group. In the authors' view, these observations (excessive amounts of n-6 PUFA in the one instance and deficiency of n-3 PUFA in the other) could cause chronic inflammation and endothelial dysfunction of microvasculature. Thus, theoretically, a more balanced fatty acid intake could help to prevent dementia.

Similarly, in the Rotterdam study, increased total fatty acid intake appeared to be a risk factor for dementia (RR 2.4; CI 1.1, 5.2), as did increased saturated fatty acid intake (RR 1.9; CI 0.9, 3.2).[4] High consumption of fish, an important source of n-3 unsaturated fatty acids, decreased the risk of dementia (RR 0.4; CI 0.2, 0.9). Similar results were also observed in the PAQUID study[5] and in the Zutphen study, high fish consumption tended to be inversely correlated with decline of cognitive function (RR 0.5; CI O.2, 1.2).[6]

Pratico et al[7] studied the levels of isoprostane (a specific marker of fat peroxidation) in the plasma, urine, and cerebrospinal fluid (CSF) of 50 patients with AD, 30 patients classified as having MCI, and 40 control subjects. The level of urinary isoprostane was significantly higher in AD patients than in controls (4.6 vs 1.5 mg, $P < 0.001$), but was also higher in MCI patients than in controls (3.6 vs 1.5 mg, $P < 0.001$). Urinary isoprostane also differed significantly between AD and MCI ($P < 0.01$). Similar differences were found with plasma concentrations between AD and MCI subjects (0.61 vs 0.44, $P < 0.03$), and between MCI subjects and controls (0.44 vs 0.19, $P < 0.001$). The same correlations were found in the CSF. This work demonstrates, on a biological level, the increase of oxidative stress in AD subjects, but also in MCI. If we accept the nosological continuum of MCI–AD, this proves that oxidative brain damage occurs very early, well before the clinical phase of the disease. Measurement of urinary and plasma isoprostane would perhaps make it possible to identify, among MCI patients, those who are the most at risk of progressing dementia of Alzheimer type.

Oxidative stress and vitamins

According to the free radical hypothesis put forward above, oxidative stress appears to be a major risk factor for AD.

Vitamins A, C, and E and metals such as zinc and selenium could thus protect against AD through their antioxidant properties.[8] Data obtained from animal studies are already convincing: for example, polyunsaturated docosahexaenoic acid prevents cognitive decline in the animal model and inhibits hippocampal lesions related to oxidative stress.[9]

In humans, vitamin E deficiency is frequently observed in patients with AD.[10] Perrig et al[11] followed 442 subjects (mean age 75 years) for 22 years. The levels of vitamins A, C, and E were measured and compared with the patients' memory performance, evaluated by various tests investigating all aspects of memory function (WAIS-R, WMC, priming, and free recall). There was a close correlation between satisfactory vitamin status and preservation of good memory function.

It seems conceivable that a diet rich in or supplemented with antioxidants could be used in the prevention of AD. Sano et al[12] showed that administration of vitamin E (2000 IU/day) to subjects with AD slowed disease progression.

Morris et al[13] carried out a longitudinal study of 2889 elderly subjects (mean age 74 years) between 1993 and 2000 (mean follow-up 3.2 years), who completed a food-frequency questionnaire. The cognitive study was carried out at 3 years by neuropsychological tests (the East Boston Memory Test, the MMSE, and the Symbol Digit Modalities Test). Cognitive performance declined on average by 5 standard units per year. In subjects with the greatest intake of vitamin E, whether from foods or supplements (highest quintile), there was a 36% reduction in the rate of cognitive decline compared with subjects in the lowest quintile ($P = 0.05$). Vitamins A and C did not appear to have a protective effect.

The same group[14] also prospectively examined, under the same conditions, 815 subjects aged over 65 years who were free of AD at baseline in order to study the relationship between the development of AD and vitamin A, C, and E intake with a food-frequency questionnaire. Mean follow-up was 3.9 years. ApoE typing was carried out. The incidence of AD was evaluated from the diagnosis of a neurologist and a neuropsychologist (using the CERAD tests). By the end of the 3.9 years, 131 persons had developed AD. High vitamin E intake was correlated with a lower risk of developing AD only in non-ApoE4 subjects (incidence 4.2% in the quintile of highest vitamin E intake vs 16.7% in the quintile of lowest intake, OR 0.17; CI 0.06, 0.47). Vitamin A and C intake was not correlated with decreased risk of AD.

Engelhart et al[15] studied a population of 5395 persons aged over 55 years, free of dementia, with a mean follow-up of 6 years. Vitamin intakes were evaluated by semiquantitative food-frequency questionnaires. After 6 years, 197 cases of dementia had been diagnosed, including 146 of Alzheimer type. High vitamin C and E intake seemed to reduce the risk of AD: the relative risk (RR) between the lowest tertile of vitamin C intake (< 95 mg/day) and the highest intake tertile (> 133 mg/day) was 0.66 (CI 0.44, 1.00). Similarly, the RR of developing AD between the lowest tertile of vitamin E intake (< 10.5 mg/day) and the highest tertile (> 15.5 mg/day) was 0.57 (CI 0.35, 0.91). It should be noted that these results did not vary according to ApoE genotype. The authors also found a greater benefit in smokers, in whom flavonoids and beta-carotenes were also found to be protective factors against AD, although these were not significant in the population as a whole.

Oxidative stress and alcohol

Some teams gave their attention to the antioxidant effects of phenols, present, in particular, in the tannins of red wine, and their protective effects against AD.

In a prospective study of 3777 subjects aged over 65 years, in which incident cases of AD (diagnosed by explicit criteria) were screened at 1 and 3 years, Orgogozo et al[16] showed decreased incidence in subjects consuming 250–500 ml of red wine per day, compared with nondrinkers.

These results were confirmed by the Rotterdam study[17] of 7983 subjects aged 55 years or over who did not have dementia at baseline. After 6 years' follow-up, 197 subjects had developed dementia, including 147 of Alzheimer type. Moderate drinkers (1–3 glasses a day) had a lower risk of developing dementia than nondrinkers (RR 0.58; CI 0.38, 0.90). The protective effect was independent of the type of alcohol consumed, and was greater against vascular dementia than against AD.

Truelsen et al[18] studied a population of 1709 volunteers aged over 65 years who first took the MMSE, and then neuropsychological tests and imaging for the diagnosis of dementia if the initial score was less than 24. Eighty-three cases of dementia were diagnosed, including 40 AD. The participants all described their alcohol intake in quantity and quality. Wine consumption was an independent protective factor against dementia (OR 0.33; CI 0.13, 0.86 for weekly consumption), whether it was monthly, weekly, or daily. It was noteworthy that consumption of spirits did not affect the risk of AD. Beer appeared to be a risk factor for AD (OR 2.28; CI 1.13, 4.60 for monthly consumption). The authors concluded that wine contains substances which may reduce the incidence of dementia. This retrospective study was evidently less powerful than the Rotterdam study.

Role of the vascular component

Cholesterol and Alzheimer's disease

Cardiovascular risk factors (hypercholesterolemia, diabetes, and arterial hypertension) have been implicated by certain authors as risk factors for AD. Nutrition evidently plays an essential role in these anomalies.

In a prospective study of 1449 volunteers aged 65–79 years, in Finland, with a mean follow-up of 21 years, Kivipelto et al[19] studied among other parameters the initial total cholesterol level, systolic blood pressure, ApoE genetic typing, and the development of AD. Fifty-seven participants (4%)

were diagnosed with dementia at the follow-up visit at 11, 16, 21, or 26 years. Forty-eight fulfilled the criteria for possible AD. It should be noted that 82 participants (6.1%) were classified as MCI, but were not taken into account in the rest of the study. The results showed that elevated total cholesterol (> 6.5 mmol/l) was a risk factor for AD (OR 2.8; CI 1.2, 6.7), as was elevated systolic blood pressure (OR 2.6; CI 1.1, 6.6). Statistical analysis showed that these risk factors were independent.

Yaffe et al[20] studied the relationship between cholesterol, statin use, and cognitive function in 1037 postmenopausal women with coronary heart disease, aged under 80 years (mean age 71 years), recruited at 10 centers and followed for 4 years. Triglycerides, low-density lipoproteins (LDL), high-density lipoproteins (HDL), and total cholesterol were measured at the beginning and at the end of the study. The population was divided into quartiles for each factor. The 3MS (Modified Mini-Mental State Examination) was administered at the end of the study: patients with a score of less than 84 points (> 1.5 SD) were classified as having a definite cognitive disorder. LDL cholesterol appeared to be a risk factor for cognitive disorder after adjustment (OR 1.76; CI 1.04, 2.97), as did total cholesterol (OR 1.77; CI 1.06, 2.97). Statins appeared to protect against cognitive disorder (OR 0.67; CI 0.42, 1.05). Similarly, with the same initial LDL cholesterol level, women whose level decreased during the 4-year period had lower odds of cognitive impairment (OR 0.61; CI 0.36, 1.03) than those in whom it had increased. This team therefore considered that lowering LDL is a strategy for preventing cognitive disorder in the elderly subject.

The Rotterdam study (5386 patients) and the Zutphen study (576 patients) also found that high total cholesterol was a risk factor for dementia (RR 1.7; CI 0.9, 3.2).

While we wait for current studies to confirm the possible value of cholesterol-lowering treatment in the prevention of AD, using statins in particular, nutritional advice seems crucial in this context.

Group B vitamins and homocysteine

A relationship exists between decreased serum levels of group B vitamins and folates, and decreased cognitive function.[21,22] On a biochemical level, deficiency in B vitamins and folates leads to defective synthesis of methionine and of S-adenyl-methionine (SAM). These two molecules are essential in the metabolism of myelin, membrane phospholipids, and neurotransmitters (serotonin, dopamine, noradrenaline, and acetylcholine). Disturbances of brain metabolism related to these deficiencies in vitamins B_1, and B_6, B_{12} and in folates could explain the cognitive disturbances observed.

There is another consequence of defective synthesis of methionine and of SAM due to inadequate intake of vitamin enzyme cofactors, notably B_{12}; this is accumulation of the product, that is, homocysteine, upstream of this metabolic methylation pathway. The second metabolic pathway of homocysteine degradation by transsulfuration involves vitamin B_6 as an enzyme cofactor of cystathionine-synthetase. A deficiency of group B vitamins thus leads to accumulation of homocysteine, which seems to play a role in the decline of brain function,[23] perhaps due to its direct cytotoxic effect on the vascular endothelium. In a prospective study of 370 elderly persons in Sweden, low serum levels of folates or vitamin B_{12} doubled the risk of AD.[24]

Very interesting results were obtained in the largest and longest study carried out on the subject, the Framingham study[25] in which 1092 subjects without dementia (667 women, 425 men; mean age 76 years) were followed for a mean of 8 years, with an MMSE every 6 months and a battery of neuropsychological tests yearly. Measurements of plasma homocysteine, vitamins B_6 and B_{12} and folates were carried out, as well as ApoE typing. At the end of follow-up, 111 patients had developed dementia, among them 83 of Alzheimer type. The results showed that elevated plasma homocysteine above 14 µmol/l was an independent risk factor for AD (RR 1.9; CI 1.3, 2.8). In addition, this relation was strong and proportional, since the team of Seshadri et al found that a 5 µmol/l increase in plasma homocysteine increased the risk of AD by 40% ($P < 0.001$), with no effect of sex or age. However, serum levels of vitamins B_6 and B_{12} and folates did not seem to be independent risk factors. Elevated plasma homocysteine thus seems to be significantly involved in the development and also the progression of AD.

In a study of 43 patients with AD and 37 control subjects, Miller et al[26] found that it was the 'vascular' subgroups (history of coronary heart disease, transient ischemic episodes, or stroke) who had elevated plasma homocysteine, both in the control group without AD and in the group with dementia. They concluded that elevated plasma homocysteine was related only to the vascular lesions, and not to AD. However, they considered it probable that this microlesional vascular component was primarily responsible for the aggravation of the disease.

However, McIlroy et al[27] found that elevated plasma homocysteine was a risk factor for AD independently of vascular risk factors and of nutritional status. So the debate continues.

In the population of the Rotterdam study, Prins et al[28] examined the links between plasma homocysteine and cognitive performances in nondemented subjects. In the 1077 subjects, elevated plasma homocysteine was correlated with lower scores on neuropsychological tests of psychomotor skills (–0.26; CI–0.37, –0.14), memory (–0.13; CI –0.27, 0.01) and overall cognitive functioning (–0.20; CI –0.30 , –0.11) between patients in the highest quintile (> 14 µmol/l) and those in the lowest quintile (< 8.5 µmol/l).

Also noteworthy is an interesting article by McCaddon et al[29] who affirm that for biochemical reasons the pharmaceutical forms of vitamin B_{12} that are currently available (adenosylcobalamine and methylcobalamine) cannot be metabolized by neurons subjected to oxidative stress, since they must be broken down in order to be internalized.

Although it has no real connection with the mechanisms we have previously mentioned, a study on coffee presented astonishing results. Caffeine, known for its psychostimulatory properties, may have long-term beneficial effects on cognitive function in chronic consumers. This emerges from a retrospective study by Johnson-Kozlow et al[30] of 1628 persons (890 women, 638 men; mean age 73 years). Their coffee consumption was evaluated by questionnaire. Cognitive function was assessed by a battery of 12 standardized tests. After adjustment, women (only) who were heavy coffee drinkers performed significantly better on six of 12 tests ($P < 0.05$). If the coffee was decaffeinated, the result was no longer positive. These results should be taken with caution.

In conclusion, it is now high time to set up large interventional studies with the aim of validating these hypotheses. Some are already underway, with vitamin E in MCI, or with *Ginkgo biloba* extract (EgB 761), in the USA and in Europe. Others are in preparation. Such studies are very cumbersome and costly to set up, but they appear to be indispensable as long as we are confronted with a disease as devastating as AD; if nutritional intervention is found to have the impact we hope for, it will be put into general use, fulfilling the aim of prevention that is so sought after in modern health systems. A policy of nutritional advice similar to that proposed to patients at risk of cardiovascular disease could then be envisaged.

References

1. Sparks DL, Hunsaker JC, Scheff SW et al. Cortical senile plaques in coronary artery disease, aging and Alzheimer's disease. Neurobiol Aging 1990; 11:601–607.

2. Luchsinger J, Tang MX, Shea S et al. Caloric intake and the risk of Alzheimer disease. Arch Neurol 2002; 59:1258–1263.

3. Otsuka M, Yamaguchi K, Ueki A et al. Similarities and differences between Alzheimer's disease and vascular dementia from the viewpoint of nutrition. Ann N Y Acad Sci 2002; 977:155–161.

4. Breteler MM. Vascular risk factors from Alzheimer's disease: an epidemiologic perspective. Neurobiol Aging 2000; 21:153–160.

5. Barbeger-Gateau P, Letenneur L, Deschamps V. Fish, meat, and risk of dementia. BMJ 2002; 325:932–933.

6. Kalmijn S. Fatty acid intake and the risk of dementia and cognitive decline: a review of clinical and epidemiological studies. J Nutr Health Aging 2000; 4:202–207.

7. Pratico D, Clark C, Liun F et al. Increase of brain oxidative stress in mild cognitive impairment. Arch Neurol 2002; 59:972–976.

8. Ortega RM, Requejo AM, Andres P et al. Dietary intake and cognitive function in a group of elderly people. Am J Clin Nutr 1997; 66:803–809.

9. Akbar M, Kim HY. Protective effects of docosahexaenoic acid. J Neurochem 2002; 82:655–665.

10. Jeandel C, Nicolas MB, Dubois F et al. Lipid peroxidation and free radical scavengers in Alzheimer's disease. Gerontology 1989; 35:275–282.

11. Perrig WJ, Perrig P, Stahelin HB et al. Relation between antioxidants and memory performance in the old and very old. J Am Geriatric Soc 1997; 45:718–724.

12. Sano M, Ernesto C, Thomas RG et al. A controlled trial of selegiline, alpha-tocopherol, or both as treatment for Alzheimer's disease. N Engl J Med 1997; 336:1216–1222.

13. Morris MC, Evans D, Bienias J et al. Vitamin E and cognitive decline in older persons. Arch Neurol 2002; 59:1125–1132.

14. Morris MC, Evans D, Bienias J et al. Dietary intake of antioxidant nutrients and the risk of incident Alzheimer disease in a biracial community study. JAMA 2002; 287:3230–3237.

15. Engelhart MJ, Geerlings MI, Ruitenberg A et al. Dietary intake of antioxidants and risk of Alzheimer disease. JAMA 2002; 287:3223–3229.

16. Orgogozo JM, Dartigues JF, Lafont S et al. Wine consumption and dementia in the elderly. Rev Neurol 1997; 153:185–192.

17. Ruitenberg A, van Swieten JC, Witteman J et al. Alcohol consumption and risk of dementia: the Rotterdam study. Lancet 2002; 359:281–286.

18. Truelsen T, Thudium D, Gronbaek D et al. Amount and type of alcohol and risk of dementia. Neurology 2002; 59:1313–1319.

19. Kivipelto M, Helkala EL, Laakso M et al. ApoE4, elevated midlife total cholesterol level, and high midlife systolic blood pressure are independent risk factors for late-life Alzheimer disease. Ann Intern Med 2002; 137:149–155.

20. Yaffe C, Barrett E, Lin F et al. Serum lipoprotein levels, statin use, and cognitive function in older women. Arch Neurol 2002; 59:378–384.

21. Riggs KM, Spiro A, Tucker K et al. Relations of vitamin B_{12}, vitamin B_6, folate, and homocysteine to cognitive performance in the normative aging study. Am J Clin Nutr 1996; 63:306–314.

22. La Rue A, Koehler KM, Wayne SJ et al. Nutritional status and cognitive functioning in a normally aging sample. Am J Clin Nutr 1997; 65:20–29.

23. Joosten E, Lesaffre E, Riezler R et al. Is metabolic evidence for vitamin B_{12} and folate deficiency more frequent in elderly patients with Alzheimer disease? J Gerontol A Biol Sci Med Sci 1997; 52:76–79.

24. Wang HX, Wahlin A, Basun H et al. Vitamin B_{12} and folate in relation to the development of Alzheimer's disease. Neurology 2001; 56:1188–1194.

25. Seshadri S, Beiser A, Selhub J et al. Plasma homocysteine as a risk factor for dementia and Alzheimer's disease. N Engl J Med 2002; 346:476–483.

26. Miller JW, Green R, Mungas DR et al. Homocysteine, vitamin B_6, and vascular disease in AD patients. Neurology 2002; 58:1471–1475.

27. McIlroy SP, Dynan KB, Lawson JT et al. Moderately elevated plasma homocysteine and risk for stroke, vascular dementia, and Alzheimer disease in Northern Ireland. Stroke 2002; 33:2351–2356.

28. Prins ND, Den Heijer T, Hofman A et al. Homocysteine and cognitive function in the elderly. Neurology 2002; 59:1375–1380.

29. McCaddon A, Regland B, Hudson P et al. Functional vitamin B_{12} deficiency and Alzheimer disease. Neurology 2002; 58:1395–1399.

30. Johnson-Kozlow M, Kritz-Silverstein D, Barrett E et al. Coffee consumption and cognitive function among older adults. Am J Epidemiol 2002; 156:842–850.

Index